The
Recognition and Management
of
Food Allergy
in
Children

The
Recognition and Management
of
Food Allergy
in
Children

Edited by A. J. Franklin

Consultant Paediatrician,
St. John's Hospital, Chelmsford, England

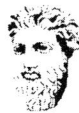

The Parthenon Publishing Group
International Publishers in Science & Technology

Casterton Hall, Carnforth,
Lancs, LA6 2LA, U.K.

120 Mill Road, Park Ridge,
New Jersey, U.S.A.

Published in the UK by
The Parthenon Publishing Group Limited
Casterton Hall, Carnforth,
Lancs, LA6 2LA, England

ISBN 1–85070–142–3

Published in the USA by
The Parthenon Publishing Group Inc.
120 Mill Road,
Park Ridge,
New Jersey 07656, USA

ISBN 0–940813–22–X

Printed in Great Britain by
Butler & Tanner Ltd, Frome and London

Contents

List of Contributors

M. K. BASU
Dept. of Oral Pathology
The Dental School
St. Chad's Queensway
BIRMINGHAM B4 6NN

C. BLAIR
Old Church Hospital
Romford
ESSEX

J. BROSTOFF
Dept of Immunology
Middlesex Hospital
4 Mortimer Street
LONDON

M. J. BRUETON
Dept. of Child Health
Charing Cross and Westminster Medical
    School
Westminster Children's Hospital
Westminster
LONDON

A. M. EDWARDS
Medical Director
Fisons Pharmaceuticals Ltd
12 Derby Road
Loughborough
LEICESTER LE11 0BB

A. J. FRANKLIN
St John's Hospital
Wood Street
Chelmsford
ESSEX CM2 9BG

S. LINGAM
Wolfson Centre
Mecklenburgh Square
LONDON WC1

J. M. LITTLEWOOD
St. James' Hospital
Beckett Street
Leeds
WEST YORKSHIRE LS9 7LF

R. MATTIS
Bexley Health Authority
Bexley
KENT

A. MacDONALD
Birmingham Children's Hospital
Ladywood
Middleway
BIRMINGHAM B16 8DT

L. M. McEWEN
Weir View
Wargrave Road
Henley-on-Thames
OXON

I. MENZIES
Dept. of Child Psychology
University of Dundee
Ninewells Hospital
Dundee
SCOTLAND

D. RAPP
State University of New York
1421 Colvin Boulevard
Buffalo
New York 14223
U.S.A.

M. SAVAGE
Abbey Chase
Bridge Road
Chertsey
SURREY

G. SUPRAMANIAM
Watford General Hospital
Vicarage Road
Watford
HERTS WD1 8HB

J. THORN
Housewife and mother,
Chatham
KENT

D. G. WRAITH
The Churchill Hospital
Headington
OXFORD OX3 7LJ

Foreword

The double-blind crossover trial (or double-cross and blind you trial!) has been accepted by modern medicine as the way to prove that any particular treatment is effective. This is a view heavily sponsored by the pharmaceutical industry, not least because this form of trial is particularly appropriate to assessing new drug regimens.

The managements described in this book do not lend themselves to such trials, nor do they provide a motive for large-scale research sponsorship. The authors are therefore faced with presenting an approach for which they would largely admit that there is a paucity of irrefutable scientific 'evidence'.

How can this be justified when the whole panoply of medicine has been erected to protect the unsuspecting populace from charlatans and quacks who sell ineffective remedies and nostrums? To respond to this valid criticism it is fair to refer to our medical forefathers who had to develop treatments without the support of statisticians. Naturally there were errors such as bloodletting and leeches (recently enjoying a comeback to the medical scene), but there were successes such as digitalis, quinine and thyroid extract.

My own experience, and that of many of the authors in this book, is that I came to appreciate the importance of diet in the management of certain symptoms after having an opportunity to listen to parents' detailed descriptions of what was happening to their children. We need always to be aware that certain patients will not be telling us the 'whole truth', with the Munchausen syndrome as the extreme result of this. It does, however, seem that we have developed an inclination to disregard everything that we are told as being unreliable, an approach which would seem to underrate the intelligence of our patients. Again, our medical forefathers were able to spend more time listening to what they were being told, which enabled them to filter out the inaccurate information and still learn from what the patient was saying.

On a more pragmatic point, we must remain aware that if the medical profession does not offer to help with dietary management, our patients will undoubtedly seek help elsewhere. They are then at risk of receiving unreliable diagnoses at considerable cost. We do not have conventional medical solutions for conditions such as severe eczema and asthma, severe hyperactivity, disordered concentration, severe migraine, etc., all of which are very difficult conditions for our patients to live with and for which they will seek any help. We can try to assist them with diet, but even if this is not effective we shall still be there to support our patients and offer them other, more conventional, remedies.

May I therefore commend to readers that, having read these chapters, you return to some of your 'difficult' cases and review their history from the perspectives suggested by the authors. In some instances you may feel that there is some relevance to the statement 'you are what you eat'.

For the future, we may see the increased use of an 'audit' of a total approach to patient care, rather than the double-blind trial as a means of assessing the usefulness of our work.

M. Tettenborn
Paediatrician

Introduction

A. J. Franklin

An increasing interest in allergy in general and food allergy in particular in recent years, especially amongst mothers, has left the medical profession sometimes sceptical, sometimes bewildered and frequently unable to respond through lack of knowledge. Allergy may be the fashion of the decade, or simply a new name for an old phenomenon, but it is generally agreed that allergic diseases are increasing. They often start in the young and affect many organ systems. Unlike many causative agents in medicine, many different allergens may produce the same clinical condition, or the same allergen may produce many different symptoms – which leads to confusion. Clinical allergists, usually highly motivated and self-taught, are aware of this diversity but within it can detect common patterns which allow them to offer logical treatment. To represent this complexity, imagine a factory trying to tool-up and computerise the control of many products and functions – extracting raw materials needed in the right amounts and storing some of the less readily available materials in order to keep the production line going. This may be particularly difficult when those delivering the raw materials have little idea of what is required or the quantities and frequency of the materials needed to supply the end product.

However, the body has to go on doing this for years and years without stopping for a scheduled reconditioning or restocking time. Noxious agents and harmful organisms need to be effectively eliminated; both trace elements and bulk raw materials must be selected from the moving belt of foods passing through the gut and the unwanted safely eliminated. Repair on the job has to be provided for, together with a carefully coordinated communications system that enables the whole to function as one organism. In children this may be further complicated by growth. It should not be surprising, therefore, that when subjected to certain kinds of stress the machine temporarily malfunctions. Miriam Polunin has pointed out that in Britain it is normal for ordinary people to rate themselves only 60–80% healthy and that the prevalence of certain diseases is related to a particular life-style and diet, but that these can change if people change their life-style and diet without having to travel halfway across the world. The industrial revolution, two major European wars, easy travel, the technological revolution and the changing concepts of social life and opportunity which these, and education, have brought have radically changed in the last century and are still changing our way of life. Violence is not new in the world but we are much more worried about violence in, or to children and young people and find it puzzling that children seem to lose control so easily. New diseases arise from time to time and a careful analysis of historical records shows this to be true, if not in the incidence of the disease, then certainly in its prevalence.

Our bodies are being required to change too rapidly, and this may be one of the major factors in the apparent health breakdown. We do not, even in one lifetime, have time to adapt to change, much less in the space of twenty-five years. The experience of Francis Pottinger* and his laboratory cats in the 1930s, as well as McCarrison's observations in India, should make us stop and think again about food as a source of ill health.

Since the Second World War we have lived through an era which, starting with antibiotics, has seen a pharmaceutical revolution in medicine. New drugs can be designed in the laboratory to produce certain effects, even though field testing has shown up to 10% of people can react abnormally to any given drug. We have come to rely on this form of medicine to control all undesirable effects and diseases, forgetting that a basic supply of nutrients and immunological mechanisms can be of equal importance and may have more far-reaching effects, because the state of the organism may modify the effect that the drug or micro-organism has upon it, for example, vitamin status and thalidomide on neural tube defects and skeletal structure.

Food is very important to children. They spend a great deal of time and effort (later money also) on food and drink – or sometimes trying to avoid it! If individual hypersensitivity to, or the misappropriation of, food could be responsible for some of the problems of both children and adults, it is surely worth looking into in the light of what is known about its effects.

This book does not attempt a formal assessment of the mechanism of digestion and absorption of food – there are many texts which deal with this both at the level of school biology or more advanced gastro-enterology. Neither does it attempt to explain the steadily unravelling mysteries of the immune system, but will make certain assumptions about what is generally recognised in these areas of medicine. The purpose is to provide a practical handbook for field workers, general practitioners, school doctors, health visitors and nurses who have to deal with the day-to-day problems in families where children's health may be affected by the food they are or are not consuming. More scientific accounts can be found in at least three other texts (see Appendix 4).

The chapters in this book are based on talks given at two-day conferences held in London and Birmingham in 1985 and 1986, sponsored by Wyeth Post Graduate Education Department, for Allergy International, a small

---

* Pottinger found that feeding laboratory cats on a crude artificial diet of cooked meat and milk led to a series of changes in physique and function which increased over five generations. The cats developed skeletal and hormonal changes, allergies, diminished sexual differences, congenital malformations in their offspring and finally total infertility. The changes were reversed over another five generations when the survivors were fed again on a natural raw food diet.

professional group whose aim was to increase knowledge of allergy diagnosis and treatment for those in closest contact with allergic children. The author has drawn freely on these presentations and is indebted to the original speakers for permission to use their material. Each of the original speakers at the conferences is actively involved in dealing with patients presenting with food-related problems and has much practical experience in this field. I hope the reader will find the contributions helpful in trying to solve some of the problems that seem to derive from that 'other working' of the body that so few of us were taught about when we started learning medicine but which present with increasing frequency in today's paediatric practice.

FOOD INTOLERANCE

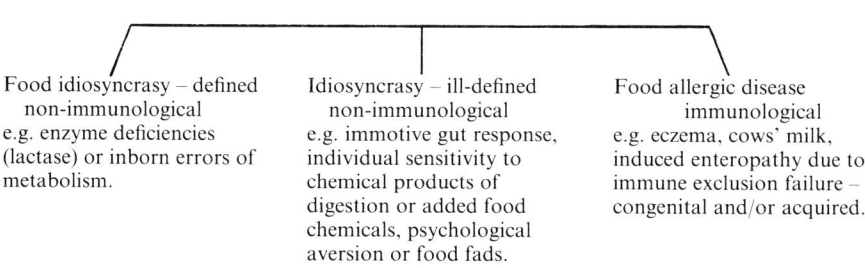

Food idiosyncrasy – defined non-immunological e.g. enzyme deficiencies (lactase) or inborn errors of metabolism.

Idiosyncrasy – ill-defined non-immunological e.g. immotive gut response, individual sensitivity to chemical products of digestion or added food chemicals, psychological aversion or food fads.

Food allergic disease immunological e.g. eczema, cows' milk, induced enteropathy due to immune exclusion failure – congenital and/or acquired.

Figure 1   Scheme for considering food allergy and intolerance (modified from Soothill, 1982).

Food allergy is starting to be recognised more often and the diagnosis of food intolerance is becoming more respectable. From a scientific point of view we still have a long way to go but this should not deter us from making clinical diagnoses now in order to meet the needs of our patients. If we fail, either they and their families will go on suffering and complaining or they will take themselves elsewhere. It is my hope that this small book will make it easier to recognise the effects of food intolerance (whatever the mechanism) and so apply an appropriate treatment to the patient.

A. J. Franklin
May 1988

1

Basic mechanisms – an overview

J. Brostoff

The diagnosis of food allergy is a problem because it is based on clinical criteria. Although in many areas of medicine a diagnosis can be confirmed or refuted by the use of appropriate laboratory tests, this is not the case with allergic diseases or food intolerance. However, allergy is not the only area where this is a problem. Angina is a clinical diagnosis, essential hypertension, idiopathic thrombo-cytopaenia, functional abdominal pain, constitutional dwarfism and hyperkinetic syndrome are all clinical terms describing a disease entity which can be treated but which also covers with a cloak of ignorance our detailed understanding of aetiology or pathology.

Current concepts of food intolerance

Pharmacological or false food allergies

Several foods contain and may release during digestion pharmacological agents, such as histamine in fish or tyramine in some cheeses, which have an unpleasant effect on those who eat them. In a survey of London academic staff as many as one-third of the total number questioned were unhappy about particular foods but they were intolerant of and not allergic to these foods. Coffee contains caffeine, itself a pharmacological agent which has differing effects in different persons according to their sensitivity. Finn and Cohen showed in 1977 that the office workers' 'Saturday morning headache' could be attributed to the withdrawal of the stimulant effect of caffeine when the pattern of life changes and the intake of caffeine decreases. Other substances such as the acetanilide in rape seed oil may be toxic and if ingested may lead to lung disease (Tabuenca, 1981).

Food idiosyncracy or congenital enzyme deficiency

This may cause difficulties in digestion of some foods. It is normal for many races of the world to lose their intestinal lactase after weaning and so be

1

unable to digest milk. The Australian author Maureen Minchin states in her well referenced book *Food for Thought* (1986) that she is convinced that lactose intolerance is quite often misdiagnosed and mistreated in Australia.

Food fads

The power of suggestion can be very great, as is also the power of placebo. The greatest danger of diet addiction is malnutrition, which can be particularly serious if it is applied by a parent to a child without any real evidence that the dietary restriction is necessary.

True food allergy

A true food allergy may alter immunological reactions in relation to food ingestion. If we were to be immunised with the amount of foreign protein that we eat by any other route than by oral ingestion, we should probably not survive the ensuing reactions. Crucial to our survival is the development of oral tolerance to these large amounts of foreign protein. If we make any response at all it will be a local immune response in the gut secreting IgA and in the circulation of powerful suppressor cells suppressing the reaction to that food protein. Some sensitised children may outgrow their allergy (or their paediatrician!), so that the adult reaction may appear in a different clinical guise, while others may remain acutely sensitive for life. Sensitisation may be associated with virus infection, for example, E-B or enteroviruses, leading to a series of chronic post-viral syndromes made worse by food sensitivity. John Hunter in Cambridge has shown a similar association between food sensitivity and alterations of bacterial gut flora in postoperative women with irritable bowel syndrome. This may not be true allergy.

Tolerance also produces problems in diagnosis, particularly when using elimination and challenge diets. Goldman's criteria gave as the standard method: (1) subsidence of the symptoms after dietary elimination; (2) recurrence of the symptoms within forty-eight hours after challenge; (3) positive identical replication for three challenges. Unfortunately, it rarely works like that because in stopping the stress of continuous challenge from food in the initial diet the patient may acquire tolerance during the elimination interval, so that he is now temporarily well from either an immunological, enzymatic or pharmacological reaction. Goldman's reproducible challenge reactions have disappeared, giving rise to doubts about the nature of the original symptoms. The time gap, the quantity and the frequency, as well as the form of presentation of the challenge, may also affect the result. The 'normal' diet of some children may be very nutritionally deficient, not in calories but in important minor nutrients, and some exclusion diets may provide a restorative balance eliminating the presenting symptoms.

Recognition

For food to be identified as an aetiological agent the symptom complex of food allergic disease must be recognised, whether it presents as Crohn's disease in adults or children, epilepsy, asthma, eczema, rhinitis, dermatitis, bloody diarrhoea, or even depression. Derek Wraith was one of the first to draw attention to this (see Figure 1), when he showed several foods caused different symptoms at different time intervals in the same patient.

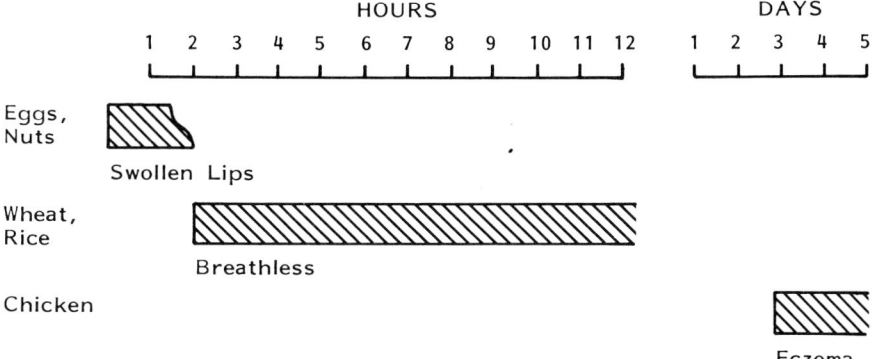

Figure 1 Time of appearance of different allergy symptoms.

Alun-Jones and John Hunter in Cambridge have shown in adults, and John Walker-Smith and Peter Milla in London in children, that Crohn's lesions can resolve just with enteral nutrition. With the more immediate anaphylactic responses the cause is obvious to the patient and does not need a positive RAST or skin-prick test to demonstrate that he has specific IgE on his mast cells, but where the symptoms are delayed the RAST and the skin-prick test may be negative and the reaction may not be IgE-mediated and the patient may not recognise the triggering factor. Irritable bowel syndrome may be compared with asthma, colic is analagous to broncho-spasm, and gas to wheezing, whereas mucous hypersecretion and mucosal oedema occur in both. The purely local mucosal response may extend into the circulation as immune complexes are released and then cause a systemic reaction.

The food man

The primary event probably occurs in the gut mucosa, where a permeability change leads to immune complexes being formed which pass into the circulation, thereby causing a form of serum sickness which is difficult to diagnose by tests unless, of course, you can directly measure the immune complexes. The patient may feel generally unwell but no specific disease follows. To demonstrate this hypothesis an egg-sensitive asthmatic patient was challenged orally by feeding egg and the asthmatic response was measured. After pre-treatment with oral sodium cromoglycate a subsequent egg challenge failed to trigger the asthmatic response. As cromoglycate is very poorly absorbed

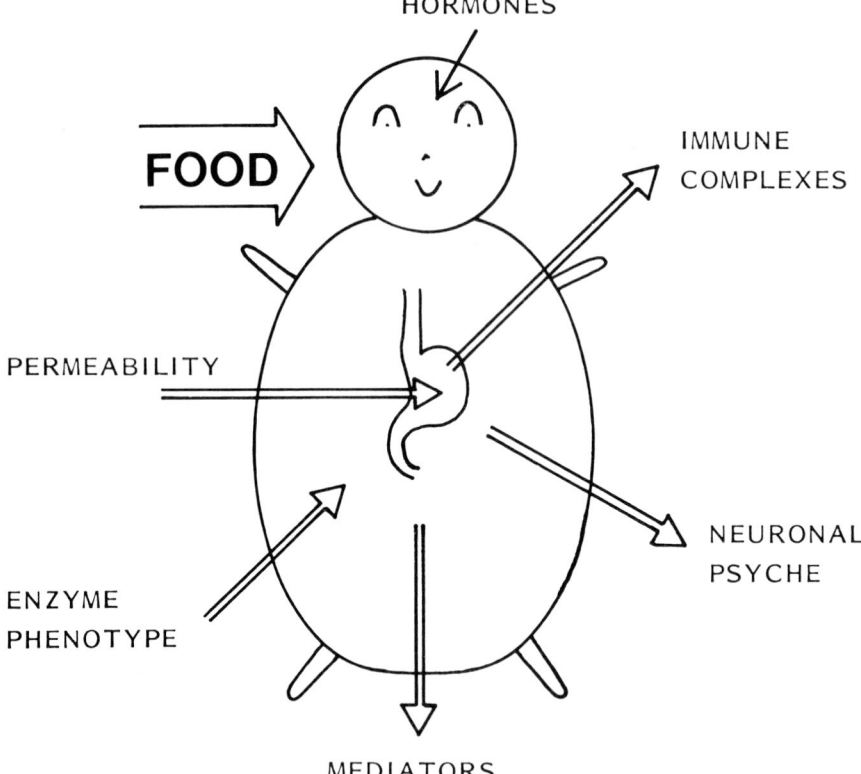

Figure 2 The Food Man.

into the circulation, the result showed that the gut was protected from the effect of the egg antigen. Sodium cromoglycate given by inhalation to the same patient failed to protect the lung from the oral egg challenge. The experiment was placebo-controlled.

In this example the target organ was the lung but it could equally have been the skin in vasculitis, the joints in rheumatoid disease, the kidney in lupus or the brain in migraine. The localisation of the complexes is a great problem not really understood by immunologists. Immune complexes with IgE considerably expand the potential for causing tissue damage. Mast cells and basophils have receptors for IgE and we now know that macrophages, eosinophils and platelets also have receptors for IgE, each producing different mediators. Activated platelets, for example, coated with IgE, effectively kill Schistosomulae in schistosomiasis. The elimination of parasites may provide a *raison d'être* for this allergic mechanism.

In our simplified model (Figure 3) we can now see that mast cells triggered by an antigen in the gut's mucosa produce mediators and increased permeability, allowing the production of immune complexes which appear in

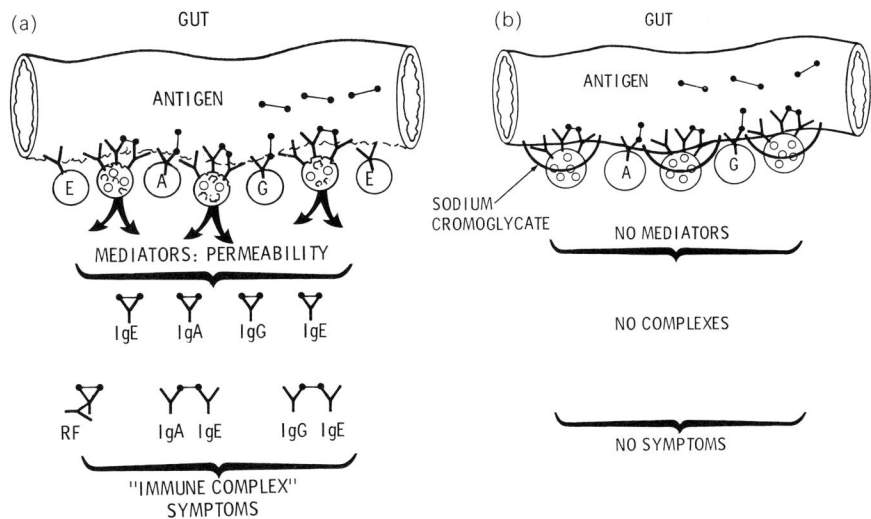

Figure 3 Suggested model for the generation of immune complexes in response to antigen (a) (food) and inhibition by sodium cromoglycate (b).

the circulation, leading to serum sickness which is difficult to diagnose but is associated with many symptoms and few signs – a characteristic of the food intolerant patient. Experimentally, in the well patient, this process can be blocked by pretreatment with sodium cromoglycate (Nalcrom), but the model may not apply to the chronically ill patient, where cromoglycate seems relatively ineffective.

The problem in the chronically ill patient is that the mucosal mast cell, which is an antigen-dependent cell, is not sensitive to sodium cromoglycate. Therefore, if a patient gets better on an exclusion diet with the antigen removed, and is then challenged with the food, after being pretreated with sodium cromoglycate or a placebo, he will now be protected by the sodium cromoglycate which originally had no effect (Figure 4). Is the diagnosis of food allergy correct, or is the gut of the chronically antigen-stimulated patient responding differently from that of the normally well patient? The difference probably lies in the different mast cell populations in these two kinds of patient. This may have practical application for children who are normally well on a restricted diet. Giving them Nalcrom before they go to parties for instance, may protect them from the foods which trigger the mast cells.

The withdrawal phenomenon

We have already commented on the power of suggestion and Goldman's attempt to be objective. An exclusion diet may be used to show the patient his symptoms will disappear if the food is not taken, but sometimes the diet has no effect because we have missed the food to which the patient is sensitive. We walk a medical tight-rope by telling the patient he may get worse before he gets better.

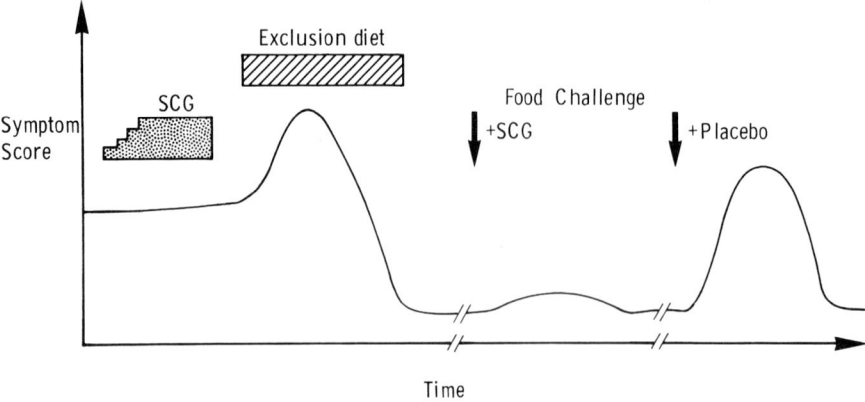

Figure 4   Effect of diet on response to sodium cromoglycate

On my theory a patient with chronic serum sickness eating large amounts of suspect foods is producing an excess of antigen in the antigen antibody complexes which makes the complexes more soluble. On an exclusion diet the amount of antigen is reduced, and the patient rises up the precipitation curve from excess antigen to excess antibody. As the amount of antigen falls, so the complexes become less soluble, the symptoms increase and the diet appears to have failed! However, a few days later the patient reaches a point on the curve where there is now an excess of antibody and the complexes are again soluble, with resolution of the symptoms – the patient feels much better (Figure 5). There are data to show that this can happen in patients with chronic arthralgia, where during withdrawal their precipitatable immune complexes first increase and then decrease. Therefore, whether the withdrawal reaction is pharmacological, endorphin-mediated, immune complex-mediated or psychologically mediated, it is a real phenomenon.

Mediators

We have already seen that mediators are important in promoting the allergic reaction. Unfortunately, not much is known about the mediators released in the human gut, but we do know that there are at least two kinds of either preformed or newly formed mediators from mast cells, known as leucotrienes and prostaglandins. There are some experiments which show that both aspirin and other non-steroidal anti-inflammatory drugs will block so-called allergic reactions, possibly by blocking some metabolic product of arachidonic acid, that is, in the cyclo-oxygenase pathway, and that if you can block pro-staglandin production by one family of mast cells that may be a way of blocking the whole reaction. However, there are other problems with mediators. Data collected by Bjarnason and Peters (1984) have shown that if you have a damaged ('leaky') gut, then mediator responses may be worse. Alcohol is a very good way of increasing gut permeability. The non-steroidal anti-inflammatory drugs also increase gut permeability. It may therefore be

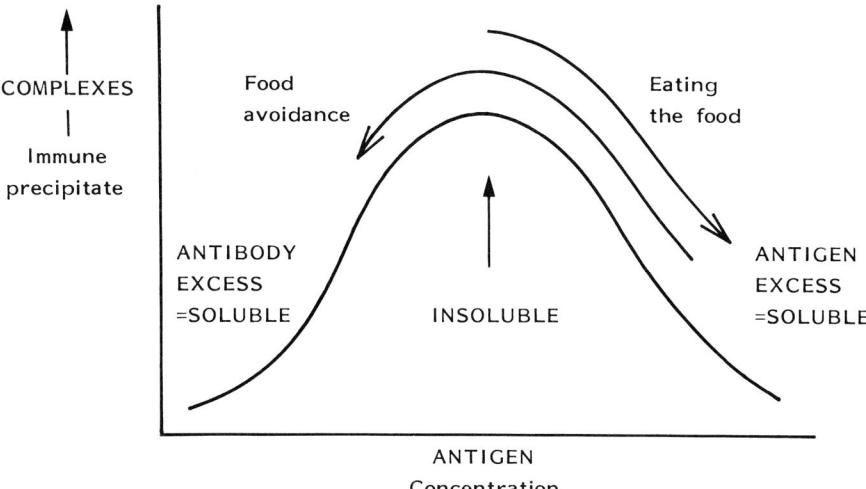

Figure 5 The relationships between antigen, antibody and immune complexes in the production of food withdrawal symptoms

possible to reduce food intolerance reactions by avoiding non-steroidal anti-inflammatory drugs and alcohol. Another unexplained paradoxical reaction is that in some cases aspirin may protect against an allergic reaction, whereas in other cases patients may be made worse by aspirin.

A good example of some enhanced effects is described by Maulitz (1979). He described a marathon runner who could run a full course provided he did not eat oysters and shrimps, because he was known to be allergic to them, but if he did eat them he could only reach about 8 km before developing an urticarial reaction and becoming breathless. This is not simple allergy but a food-related, exercise-induced urticaria/anaphylaxis syndrome in which there is a complicated inter-relationship between food allergy, exercise, mediator release and the clinical reaction which is urticaria (Figure 6).

Endorphins and addiction

Endorphins are endogenous opiates which protect the organism from pain and stress. Sometimes the newborn baby is protected by having very high levels at birth. Goetzel (1984) has introduced the concept that in response to noxious stimuli our afferent nerve fibres release a substance which forces mast cells to produce leucotrienes and histamine, which introduces the idea of the psyche being integrated into the immune system and may be producing an 'allergic reaction'. On the other hand, recently bereaved patients can be shown to have depression of lymphocyte activity; as the depression associated with bereavement improves, so the lymphocytes become more active again. Other data suggest that activated lymphocytes may produce immunoreactive ACTH, immunoreactive TRH and immunoreactive LH, so that activated lymphocytes can produce hormones as well, and in turn hormones can have effects themselves on lymphocytes and mast cells. All bodily systems are

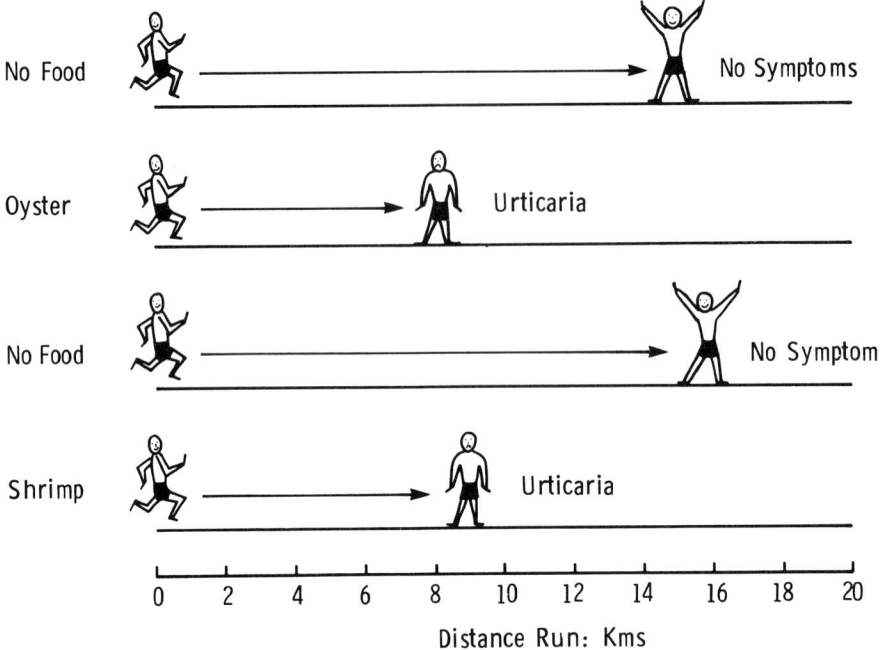

Figure 6 The effect of exercise on food allergy (reproduced from Maulitz *et al.*, 1979)

integrated, and it is important for the allergist to look at the whole person and not simply at individual systems.

Endorphins are produced in the body, but there are some compounds produced in some common foods which closely resemble endorphins, having only a few amino-acid differences in their structure. Such compounds, for example produced by the digestion of wheat and milk, are basically hormones and it is interesting to note that some food intolerant patients are indeed 'hooked' on certain foods. This would appear to be true addiction and not an immunological response after all. A further observation in food-intolerant patients is that of weight fluctuation. Hypothetically, endorphins are known to alter anti-diuretic hormone production in the rat, and in pilot studies patients who are put on the wrong diet and subjected to a waterload test retain far more water than when they are on a diet excluding milk and wheat. The difference is in excess of half a litre in an experiment in which a 20 ml per kilo waterload is given to a person weighing 50–60 kg. This is a reasonably reliable and reproducible test which suggests that perhaps some food reactions are hormonally mediated.

The 'Plastic Rose Syndrome'

One of the commonest criticisms of patients who claim a food allergy are that these are psychologically disturbed people. A simplistic conditioning view would be that if a patient is allergic to roses and sneezes when shown a

8

plastic rose then allergy is all in the mind! Even the sceptics might find it difficult to imagine a psychologically allergic guinea pig but an experiment described in *Science* has shown that there is a relationship between the mind and the immune system. Guinea pigs were immunised with a foreign protein (albumin) to produce the kind of antibody that would release histamine when they were further challenged. Starting four weeks later and for ten weeks, at weekly intervals the animals were then challenged with either antigen or placebo and at the same time they were given a smell for three seconds at the nose. They used either a sulphurous or a fishy smell on cottonwool as a conditioning response. They therefore produced three types of animal, a conditional animal, an animal that is immunised and conditioned, and another animal that isn't immunised but is conditioned. The question to be asked is whether one could produce an allergic response similar to the original antigen but only by the smell, and it was shown that when the right conditioning stimulus was applied, that is, the smell (and not the antigen), these animals released a large amount of histamine. The antigen released the same amount of histamine as the conditioning smell but the irrelevant conditioning smell released nothing. The experimenters have produced an animal that has been conditioned by smell to release the same amount of histamine as the antigen that caused the original immune response. They also showed that a second conditioning stimulus gave a slightly weaker response, which is what one would expect, but it really does raise the question about the relationship of the psyche to the immune system to a completely new plane of thinking.

In the real world allergic patients may also be conditioned to a variety of environmental stimuli. For example, a child sitting at the table with his parents may be undergoing a powerful conditioning stimulus. Going out into the world, if one is agoraphobic, may be a powerful conditioning stimulus and it may be that these conditioning stimuli relate to an allergic priming mechanism. It may be that without the priming one does not get the conditioned stimuli, but the data do show that one learns to produce histamine without the antigen, and this raises a lot of questions in relation to patients. In terms of treatment, it might even be possible to purely psychologically recondition the patient and not bother about the allergen at all. On the other hand, if one can find and eliminate the allergen what would happen to the so-called conditioning stimuli? – would they change? It is interesting to note that in the study by Egger *et al.* (1983) on childhood migraine a number of stimuli produced migraine when the patients were on their original (bad) diets but when the food allergies had been corrected these non-specific stimuli lost their ability to provoke migraine, with the exception of perfume and cigarette smoke. Of course, these exceptions may suggest that they are, after all, specific stimuli to migraine attacks. They did show that so-called emotional factors such as loud noise totally lost their efficacy once the allergen had been removed. There remains the intriguing question: if you could recondition the patient, would he not have his allergies, or, if you removed the allergy, would he not have all those psychological problems?

References

Alun-Jones, V. *et al.* (1982). Food intolerance: a major factor in the pathogenesis of the irritable bowel syndrome. *Lancet,* **ii,** 1115

Bjarnson, I. and Oeters, T. J. (1984). In vitro determination of small intestinal permeability. *Gut,* **25,** 145–50

Egger, J., Carter, C. M., Wilson, J. and Soothill, J. F. (1983). Is migraine food allergy? A double blind controlled trial of oligo-antigenic diet treatment. *Lancet,* **ii,** 865–9

Finn, R. and Cohen, H. N. (1978). Food allergy – fact or fiction. *Lancet,* **ii,** 426–8

Goetzl (1984). Inhibition by somatostatin of the release of mediators from human basophils and rat leukaemic basophils. *J. Immunol.,* **133** (6), 3255–9

Goldman, A. S. *et. al.* (1963). Milk allergy. *Paediatrics,* **32,** 425–42

Maulitz, R. H. *et al.* (1979). Exercise induced anaphylactic reaction to shellfish. *J. Allergy Clin. Immunol.,* **63,** 433–4

Minchin, M. (1986). *Food for Thought – A Parent's Guide to Food Intolerance.* Oxford University Press

Moneret-Vautrin, D. A. (1983). In Lessof, M. H. (ed.) *False Food Allergies in Clinical Reactions to Food.* Wiley & Sons, Chichester

Russell, M., Dark, K. A. *et al.* (1984). Learned histamine release. *Science,* **225,** 733

Trabuenca, J. (1981). Toxic allergic syndrome caused by ingestion of rape seed oil denatured with aniline. *Lancet,* **ii,** 567

Wraith, D. (1982). Asthma and rhinitis. *Clin. Immunol. Allergy,* **2,** 101–12

2

Immunology of the gut in children

M. J. Brueton

This chapter considers some aspects of our current understanding of immune mechanisms in the gut, beginning with a consideration of the ways in which antigens are handled by the small bowel mucosa. Originally the primary function of the immune system was regarded as the provision of protection against foreign antigens. Later the concept of immune tolerance became important and with it an appreciation that hypersensitivity states were situations in which immunological reactions coincidentally caused tissue damage.

Mucosal immunoregulation

As was mentioned in Chapter 1, tolerance to food protein is of immense importance. As long ago as 1940 it was noticed that in specific circumstances it was impossible to demonstrate an immune response to an orally administered antigen. If a mouse was given ovalbumin intraperitoneally, one could expect the animal to develop circulating antibodies to it in due course. If the mouse had previously been exposed to ovalbumin orally, then specific circulating antibodies could not be identified; in other words oral tolerance had been induced. Many years later this phenomenon was investigated in more detail and it was found that the amount of ovalbumin given orally was quite crucial, as were the number of exposures and the timing and dose of subsequent intraperitoneal injections. This raises some immediate questions, such as how is this relevant clinically and what can we learn from understanding the mechanisms for initiating and maintaining tolerance?

This leads into the whole world of lymphocytes and the gut. The gut-associated lymphoid tissue forms a vast organ. In the small bowel mucosa there are mononuclear cells including lymphocytes, macrophages and mast cells, both in the lamina propria and in the epithelium lying between the enterocytes. The lymphocytes are involved in humoral and cellular immunity and cytotoxicity, as well as in immunoregulation. In the bowel wall there are lymphocytic aggregations, called Peyer's patches, which are reminiscent of lymph nodes but without afferent lymphatics leading into them. Under the electron microscope the enterocytes appear to be different from those in ordinary villi. They are called M cells and seem to preferentially take up antigen to allow it to be presented to sensitised lymphocytes in the Peyer's patches. Thus it is assumed that the normal immune response in the gut to a new antigen would involve lymphocyte/antigen interaction within the Peyer's patches. This inevitably means that one would suspect that if lymphocytes started to encounter antigen which had crossed the mucosa at other sites one might expect a different immunological response. There are a whole series of complicated lymphocyte circulation pathways, in which the cells leave the Peyer's patches, move to other tissues within the immune system, are processed in various sites within the reticulo endothelial system and are then released into the systemic circulation. This concept means that immuno competent effector cells will be distributed throughout the body as well as the gut, where the importance of IgA has long been recognised. Thus it is now possible to put forward more detailed immunological explanations for some of the hypersensitivity reactions which are encountered in clinical practice.

Amongst the many functions of IgA is immunoexclusion of antigen. Some animal studies and a few in man have shown that the presence of specific IgA

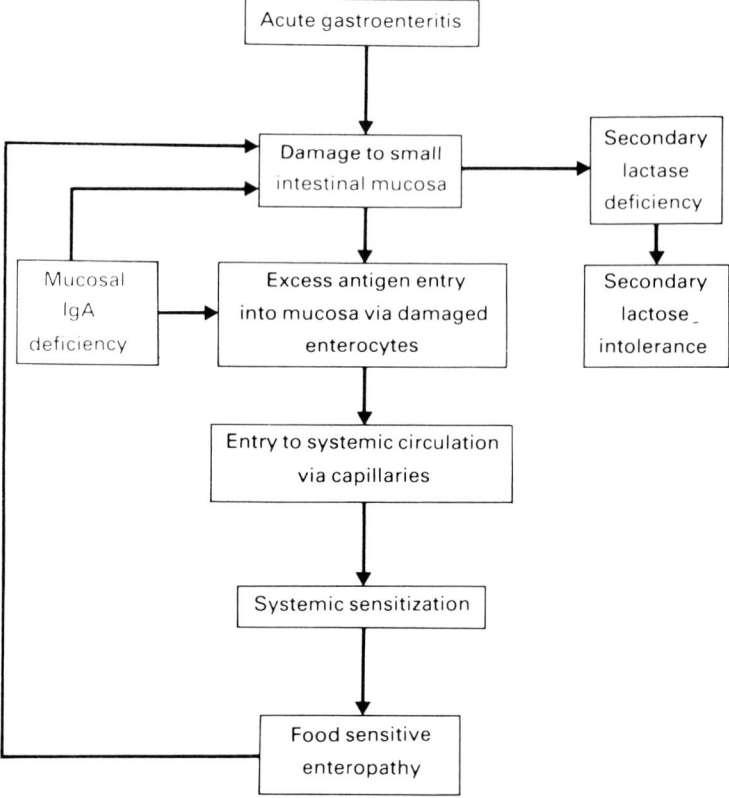

Figure 1 Hypothesis to explain relationship between gastroenteritis, food-sensitive enteropathy, IgA deficiency and secondary lactose intolerance (used with permission of W. A. Saunders & Co).

antibodies against an antigen reduces its uptake into the portal vein. In relation to oral tolerance it has now been shown that the mucosal IgA response to an antigen such as oral ovalbumin can be enhanced at the same time that suppression of systemic IgG and IgM responses to that antigen occurs. Polio immunisation, for instance, depends on local mucosal immunity rather than on the presence of circulating antibodies. This elegant arrangement of immunoregulatory pathways means that it is possible to have mucosal immunity and systemic tolerance, which clearly suggests various hypotheses concerning what might happen if something went wrong with the fine balance. There is still a good deal more to be learned about the circulation of the various T and B lymphocytes and their subsets within the gut, and between the gut and the general circulation.

In animal studies looking at lymphocyte subpopulations in various situations we found that cells expressing suppressor/cytoxicity markers predominated in neonatal rodents. Their functional involvement in suppression remains to be investigated. In malnutrition one can notice clinically that both animals and humans have problems with infection. In our animal studies the Peyer's patches showed a mature distribution of markers early on compared with the intra-epithelial lymphocytes, but in malnutrition there was a delay in the development of some of the suppressor marker positive cells. One may postulate from the animal studies that in infancy and in malnutrition there may be a maturational delay in mucosal regulation which is relevant to the ability to develop and maintain the balance between tolerance, protection and hypersensitivity. As regards the neonate, one can only begin to speculate why babies become sensitised. In addition to immaturity, the effect of large concentrations of highly antigenic proteins such as those in cow's milk could be important. If enterocytes are damaged at an early stage, proteins and other nutrients may cross the mucosa in situations where the virgin lymphocytes would not normally encounter such a stimulus and thus unusual responses could be set up. In the malnourished a reduction in IgA and changes in T cell function can all be demonstrated, with an associated deficiency in immune responsiveness; for example, marasmic children with candidiasis who gave no evidence of immune responsiveness to Candida have been shown to begin producing positive antibody and skin tests once they have been nutritionally rehabilitated. It is interesting to note how little demonstrable food allergy there is in tropical areas.

Clinical aspects

In general, there are two patterns of gastro-intestinal food allergy: one which comes on very quickly and another in which the onset is gradual and quite insidious. It is a common observation that many intolerances in infants resolve by the age of 2 years. However, if children who have suffered food intolerance are followed, some may later develop asthma, eczema, or hayfever, and some may continue to have minor enteropathies well into their school years or beyond. Cows' milk protein is the major antigen in these cases; it may be associated with small bowel enteropathies and/or colitis.

Other food proteins are also occasionally implicated, and many hypersensitivities have developed as a secondary phenomenon following gastroenteritis. It is probable that the patients were exposed to the proteins concerned during the inflammatory period at which time sensitisation took place. Confirmation would require a demonstration of jejunal biopsy changes in relation to antigen exposure and withdrawal. An interesting incidental observation is the development of enteropathies in relation to graft versus host disease in bone marrow transplantation. Here the mucosal changes that one sees resemble those encountered in cows' milk and soya protein intolerances.

Investigation

The ideal investigation would enable information to be gained about abnormalities at the mucosal level. In general we tend to measure systemic humoral responses to antigen in the blood, although we should probably be measuring local humoral and cellular responses actually in the mucosa. From the point of view of gut immunology, measuring antibodies in the serum is difficult to relate to what is actually going on locally. IgE and RAST levels are again difficult to interpret, although in very young infants there may be some correlation between high concentrations and clinical reactivity. Local mucosal studies would be more useful, but at present small bowel biopsies have some practical limitations in relation to multiple challenges. The technique is invasive and unfortunately the lesions can be patchy. More recent work using sugar probes to study permeability may be more helpful to monitor challenges, although abnormal permeability may be associated with almost normal biopsies on light microscopy. It should be borne in mind that conclusions about protein antigen permeability cannot be directly assumed from carbohydrate studies. This contrasts with coeliac disease in which jejunal biopsies show extensive histological changes. Lactase deficiency can cause difficulties, since it is a very non-specific feature of enterocyte damage. Interpreting a cow's milk challenge clinically can therefore be misleading in the presence of lactose malabsorption.

Despite the considerable amount of animal work available, our application of knowledge about mucosal immunity to the clinical management of patients is still in its infancy. In children the interaction of infection and hypersensitivity with mucosal immaturity, genetic predisposition, nutritional status and the effect of dietary and environmental factors will continue to cause confusion for many years to come.

3

The spectrum of food allergic disorders in children

S. Lingam

In this chapter we shall not attempt to differentiate between food allergy and food intolerance but shall be looking at the clinical features as they present to the physician.

Age of onset and clinical features

Some parents, asked about the onset of food allergy, will say it begins *in utero*. They tell us that their babies are very active and have increased foetal movements. They describe them as being 'stiff in the uterus' and even stiff at the time of delivery. In the neonatal period babies with food allergies seem to have a dry skin, and often cradle cap, with cracking behind the ears. They tend to be poor feeders, frequently spitting or vomiting. They are also hesitant to suck at the breast and they often have loose stools, with excessive crying. Some children suffer hiccups frequently and have colic, but, interestingly, a few become very constipated. Many of these symptoms seem to be related to milk and can be abolished or made less prominent when the type of milk feed is changed, for example by substituting soya milk feeds.

In older children facial features may be indicative of allergic sensitivity. The typical allergic faces include allergic 'shiners', oedematous swellings which occur just below and lateral to the eyes, deep creases in the lower eyelids, a bluish-grey discolouration of the orbital grooves, red noses, cheeks and ear lobes (Figure 1). They also appear to sometimes display facial mannerisms, including the so-called 'allergic salute', in which the hand is rubbed vertically upwards over the front of the nose, producing a horizontal crease two-thirds down the length of the nose (Figure 4). This is done as a result of excess mucus and irritation in the nose. Some continually twitch their noses like rabbits or they twitch the corners of their mouth. A few children also seem to develop patches of alopecia. It is noticed that once the allergies are corrected many of these features disappear.

Other children sometimes develop asthma, eczema, nasal catarrh, rhinitis and allergic conjunctivitis as a result of food allergy (Figure 5). Some children

15

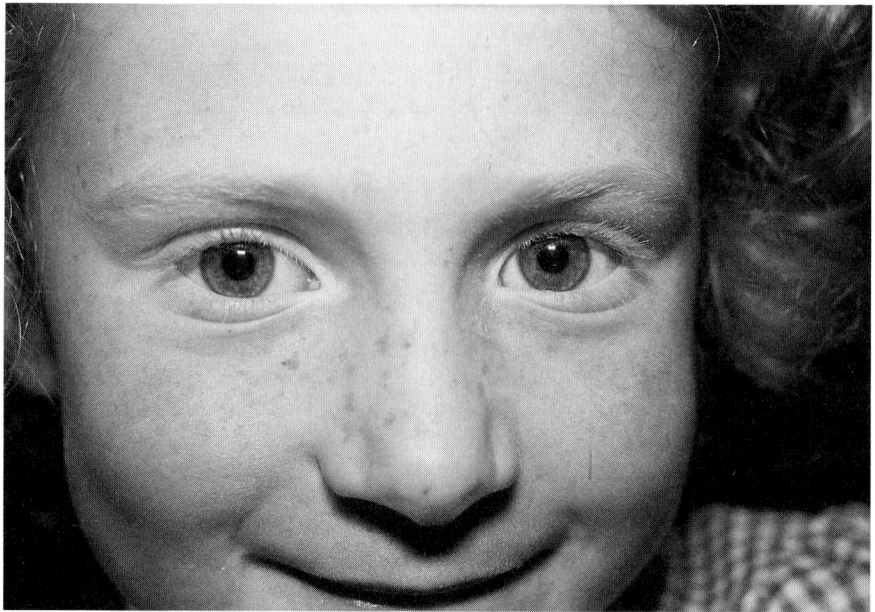

Figure 1 A typical allergic face.

have central nervous system manifestations of food allergy, exhibiting behavioural problems which I call the 'short fuse syndrome'. These are children who cannot sit still, become easily frustrated and burst into tempers. A few develop cardiac arrhythmias such as supraventricular tachycardia, with heart rates at more than 300 per minute which cause them to go into a state of panic due to severe palpitations. (I saw one child who did this as a result of eating chocolate.) In older children and adults particularly, arthritis and arthralgia may be due to food allergy, as well as night muscle cramps in the legs, which are sometimes called growing pains.

Theories of causation

One of the popular theories of causation involves the concept of a total stress load. Using a balance as a model (Figure 2), we can see that on the one side we are affected by our genetic endowment and our ability to adapt (we all have the ability to adapt but this may vary from one person to another and may be mediated by the production of adrenalin and corticosteroids), and on the other side by exposure to environmental stresses such as infection, trauma, surgery, family problems or school problems. Even pregnancy may disturb the balance, and allow sensitisation to environmental allergens to take place. Exposure to chemicals and inhalants can be important in this context, but in this chapter we are concentrating on food intolerance. Before giving examples of this I would like to make a further comment about how some children react to infection. The stress of recurrent infection may

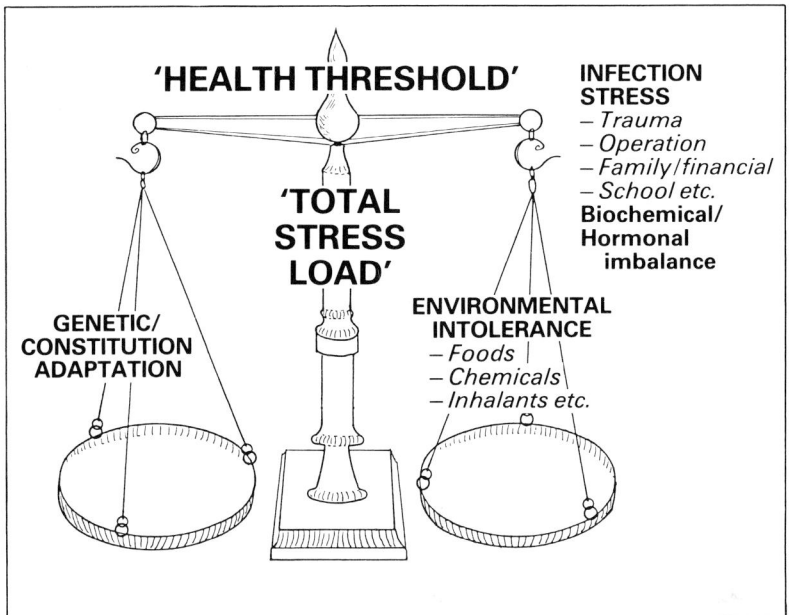

Figure 2

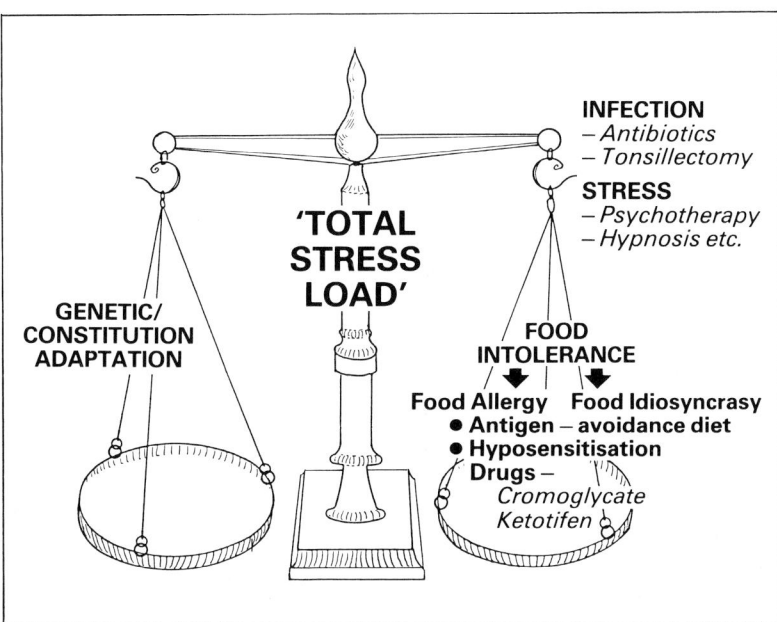

Figure 3

encourage the development of food intolerance (Figure 3). Some children's susceptibility to recurrent infection can be reduced by the continuous use of antibiotics, particularly for recurrent tonsillitis. The simple expedient of

17

tonsillectomy may help to restore the status quo. The same may also be applied to a psychological management but the allergist has the option of an antigen avoidance diet, hyposensitisation or the use of drugs. These options will be dealt with later and in the section on management.

Clinical examples

(1) Nigel was one of the youngest babies, and the first convincing one that I saw. He was born at term, with a good weight. He first attended the clinic, at the age of 5 weeks, because his weight had dropped below his birth weight. He fed poorly and was frequently sick, and it was noticed that he had been a very active baby *in utero*. His mother was atopic and had asthma. Because she was breast feeding she was advised to stop taking all dairy milk food but she phoned the next day to say she could not stop eating chocolate. Breast feeding was therefore discontinued and he was given soya formula milk, and as a result he straightaway began to thrive. Whilst weaning he was kept on a milk free/egg free diet. He still continued to refuse egg but one day did take some chocolate and was sick. Another day he had some milk and had diarrhoea. Now, at the age of 2 years, he has not yet learned to tolerate these foods but otherwise he is a healthy little boy.

(2) Laura, also an active baby *in utero*, presented with frequent coughs and colds. She was an irritable baby, always screaming and vomiting, and her parents had become exhausted by her non-stop crying. She was admitted to hospital at the age of $4\frac{1}{2}$ months and placed on a milk- and egg-free diet, these foods being replaced by a soya formula. Her colic settled and so did her screaming, and she continued to do well. At her first birthday party she drank some orange juice and on the following day her mother telephoned to say she had become very grizzly and very irritable again. She is therefore to continue with the egg-, milk-, and orange juice-free diet, at least until she is about 2 years of age.

(3) Daren was first seen at the age of 5 years with asthma. He gave a previous history of persistent loose stools and vomiting in infancy, which had led to the parents changing to various milk formulae, with no improvements. Skin prick testing showed a positive reaction to cows' milk. Milk was therefore discontinued and his subsequent asthmatic reactions were very much less severe. Further exclusion dieting revealed other foods which also contributed to his condition and on avoiding these he remains well.

(4) Jenny, a girl of 7, attended the clinic because of frequency of micturition and migrainous headache. She had no history of feeding or bowel problems but had had one febrile convulsion at the age of 1 year. The unusual feature of her diet was that she hated milk, craved eggs (had to have at least two a day) and drank a lot of orange juice. On examination she was of normal height and weight but had a little rash on her body and allergic creases and swellings under her eyes. Her IgE (immunoglobulin) levels were normal and she had no eosinophilia (high white cell count). Skin prick testing suggested she was reacting to egg, beef, chocolate, pork, tomatoes, orange, wheat and nuts. These foods were initially withdrawn. She was then put onto sodium cromoglycate, orally, and ketotifen (an antihistamine). Within two days she

had improved and was allowed home. After a short interval her polyuria returned but that seemed to be due to the fact that she had taken to drinking lemon juice and when this was withdrawn the polyuria ceased. When ketotifen was withdrawn the migraine returned. On her restrictive diet plus ketotifen she is doing well.

(5) The last example is an older child with atopic eczema from birth. She also gave a history of being active *in utero*, and having hiccups in infancy, but no feeding problems. She refused egg as a baby and had quite a lot of flatulence and colic. As a toddler she was very irritable. She slept excessively and drank excessively, mostly orange squash, and she had a salt craving. She improved greatly on a diet free from milk, peanuts, and oranges.

It is important to recognise these children who may have food intolerances but it is also very important that the child be checked by a dietitian to ensure the remaining diet is adequate, particularly in terms of vitamin and mineral intake. Self-imposed diets can easily lead to malnutrition.

Neurological symptoms

During a visit to the United States I had the opportunity to look at children aged between 2 months and 16 years (mean age $3\frac{1}{2}$ years) who were attending Dr Doris Rapp's Clinic in New York. These all had multiple symptoms. In particular, the neurological features included irritability, behaviour problems, hyperactivity, migraine, extreme fatigue and learning problems. Some children were clumsy. In addition, 80% had rhinitis, 72% had abdominal symptoms, 68% had eczema, 52% had conjunctivitis, 44% had asthma, 24% serous otitis media, and 16% enuresis. 36% had a history of food intolerance in the newborn period, another 28% during the first six months, and 10% during their first year. A total of 80% therefore gave a history of previous food intolerance. In 48% of these children there was a reluctance to take foods they were allergic to but in 32% there was excessive craving for the foods. Dr Rapp identified their food intolerance by intradermal skin testing but they were not investigated immunologically (IgE).

Most of the offending foods had actually been identified by using an antigen avoidance diet but as the children found the diet rather restrictive they were seeking further treatment such as hyposensitisation as a means of more permanently curing the problem.

Back in London the dietitian and I picked up a further sixty-two children with food related problems; forty-eight of these were on elimination diets and sixteen, in addition to diet, were on medication, either sodium cromoglycate (Intal) or ketotifen (Zaditen) or both. All the children were given vitamin B supplements and those who were totally milk-free were given calcium and zinc supplementation. A further analysis of this group of children is presented in Chapter 13.

Allergy diagnosis may be today's fashionable disease, just as syphilis and tuberculosis were in the 1920s and 1930s and collagen disease in the 1960s. I believe the possibility of allergy should also form part of the differential diagnosis of every child on whom a clear diagnosis is not forthcoming, presenting with a multisystem disorder.

19

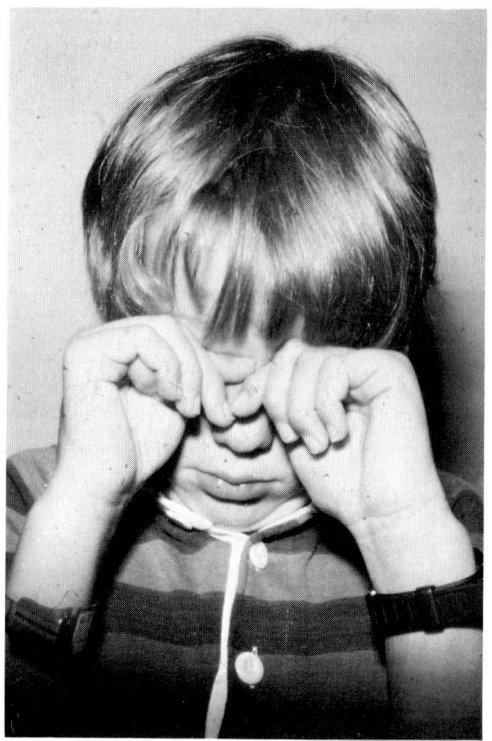
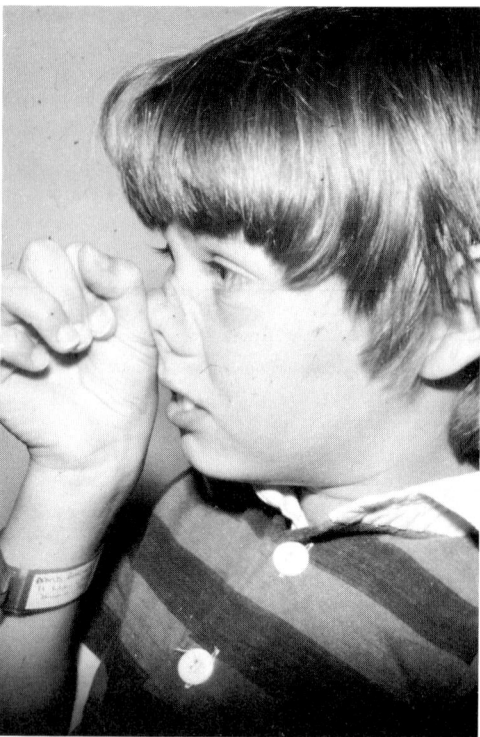

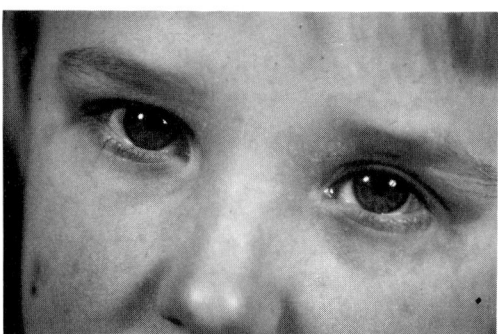
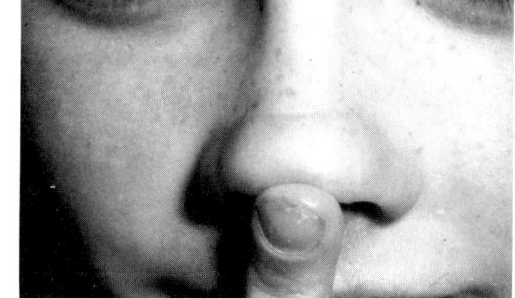

Figure 3 Allergic Conjunctivitis   **Figure 4** The Allergic Salute

Used by permission of Dr Verrier Jones, Llandough Hospital, South Glamorgan

4

Allergy of the gastro-intestinal tract

J. M. Littlewood

'Do you believe in food allergy?' This question is still asked even by professional colleagues. How can one not believe in the condition when one sees an infant covered in urticaria within seconds of taking a small quantity of egg? I suppose even the most cynical of our colleagues would accept this immediate and not infrequent type of food reaction. It is the frequency and importance of foods in the causation of a wide variety of other disorders which appears to be the main bone of contention.

Most people will be familiar with someone who has quite definite reactions to certain foods; it is rare for serious illnesses to result and the offending foods are usually avoided by the individual. However, certainly in paediatric practice, extremely serious and generally delibitating illnesses follow the ingestion of particular foods (Minford *et al.*, 1982; Littlewood and MacDonald, 1986). Thirteen years ago we investigated an infant who was failing to gain weight, coughing and vomiting, particularly in relation to feeds. For three weeks in hospital the child's symptoms and signs persisted; numerous investigations were performed, including bronchoscopy and oesophagoscopy.

Eventually, in desperation, a cows' milk-free diet was tried, and the symptoms settled within twenty-four hours. Subsequent challenges with cows' milk were followed by recurrence of symptoms until the child was 4 years of age, when he became gradually tolerant of cows' milk. This patient demonstrated the severe and chronic symptomatology which may be associated with food intolerance, particularly in young children.

Definitions

We need clear definitions to make a rational approach to this confusing and difficult subject. Firstly, there is *food intolerance*, a reproducible unpleasant reaction to a specific food or ingredient of food which is not psychologically mediated and should be reproducible under double-blind conditions. Unfortunately, this is not always possible in a busy clinic but it needs to be done to prove that the symptoms are really due to food. *Food allergy* is a similar reaction but in addition it is possible to demonstrate immunological changes, e.g., a raised specific IgE, or a positive skin test. Aversion includes both

21

psychological avoidance and conditioning in which, having taken a food you think will upset you, it commonly does, although there is no identifiable structural abnormality or immunological mechanism.

Diagnostic problems

Amongst the problems surrounding the diagnosis are those of uncritical acceptance and anecdotal evidence. There is also the problem of multiple pathology. The following is an example: two sisters aged 10 and 7 years had congenital myopathy, proved by muscle biopsy. Quite by accident, a year or two later, they were found to have cystinuria i.e., double pathology. A year or two later still their mother said that their main problem was not their muscular weakness but the chronic diarrhoea from which both had suffered from infancy. After extensive negative gastroenterological investigations including a normal jejunal biopsy, food intolerance was considered as a possible explanation. Starting a basic elimination diet led to a dramatic cessation of the diarrhoea in both girls. On subsequent challenge they had multiple food intolerance and the most important food was eggs. So here were two sisters with triple pathology.

Food allergy often seems to be associated with other conditions and should always be borne in mind when all the symptoms and signs do not fit together. The possibility of a diagnosis of food intolerance is suggested by a positive family history (at least 20% have first degree relatives with a strong history of food intolerance) and personal history of associated allergic disorders such as eczema, severe colic or vomiting in infancy. Food intolerance is a relatively common disorder of infants and young children, but as it usually is self-limiting it is unfortunate that some doctors and other health workers frequently overlook the diagnosis, accusing the mother of being neurotic or mismanaging her child. It is important to listen carefully to the parents' story; many parents will attempt a 'do-it-yourself' manipulation of the child's diet in order to try to improve the situation. Investigations are of little help in making a positive diagnosis of food intolerance but are valuable in the exclusion of alternative diagnoses. (See Chapter 12 for the correct way to manipulate the diet to reach a diagnosis.)

Jejunal biopsy

Gastroenterologists like to look at the gut in various ways. One way is to obtain a biopsy sample from the upper small bowel. Although this technique has limitations (referred to by Dr Brueton in Chapter 2) there is no doubt that mucosal changes associated with food intolerance do occur, and the demonstration of these changes in relation to food challenges has allowed all but the most cynical paediatricians in this country to accept the concept of cows' milk protein intolerance. Important studies involving serial biopsies have been reported by Professor John Walker-Smith and his colleagues (Walker-Smith et al., 1978). Not only gluten, but cows' milk, soya, rice and chicken have all produced changes in the intestinal villi of the upper small bowel. Repeat sampling shows that the villi are flat at initial presentation, when the offending food is still being taken, that they grow when the food is removed from the diet and that after rechallenge with the food they again become abnormal. This important investigation confirms the immunological damage which occurs as a result of food but it is not, of course, a practical method of investigation for every child suspected of food intolerance.

Which foods?

In our list of suspect foods milk, wheat and eggs are the most important and similar to the findings in Professor Lessof's series in adults (Minford *et al.*, 1982; Lessof *et al.*, 1980). Professor Lessof's adults do, however, seem to be more often atopic than the children.

Cows' milk intolerance is common in babies referred to my clinic. By that I mean that a number of babies are improved by putting them onto a soya or hydrolysed casein formula, though some people would claim only 1 or 2% of babies have significant symptoms due to the ingestion of cows' milk protein. Breast fed babies often have worse symptoms when their mothers are drinking cows' milk, for it has been shown that cows' milk proteins pass from the gut into the circulation and are excreted in the breast milk (Figure 1). The amounts are small compared with those imbibed by bottle fed babies

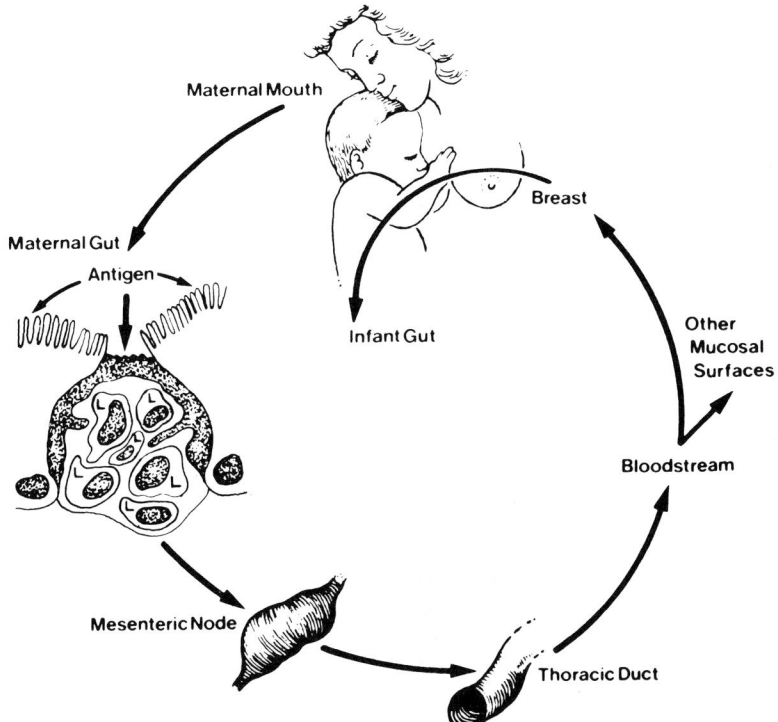

Figure 1 Circulation of possible food antigens. (Adapted from a figure courtesy of Dr Dammacco, Italy)

but the effect is greater because of the mechanisms mentioned by Dr Brostoff in Chapter 1. If a baby at the age of 2 or 3 months, after the very first – to the mother's knowledge – drink of cows' milk, develops a rash, this may not be due to sensitisation from a previous bottle feed of cows' milk slipped in soon after birth by a midwife but, more likely, to gradual sensitisation through the allergen in the mother's breast milk. It seems very unfair that the most conscientious mothers who diligently breast feed their babies may actually observe the most terrible allergic reactions in them.

Failure to thrive and infant colic

Progress charts often help to identify a child with food intolerance who is failing to progress along the normal percentile lines. In a typical case a baby with severe three-month colic, a history of poor feeding and frequent vomiting would show a rapid rise in weight gain when cows' milk was withdrawn and a soya formula substituted. Frequently such a child would be able to tolerate cows' milk quite normally by the age of 18 months. We probably now have several hundred examples like this (Figure 2). There is increasing evidence that three-month colic is related to ingestion of cows' milk protein in a significant proportion of babies. A recent study on breast fed babies by Jakobsson and Lindberg (1983) showed that when the mothers of colicky infants excluded cows' milk in a professional manner (i.e., removed from their diet all foods containing cows' milk) the infants' colic was relieved in a significant proportion. A recent study of formula fed infants by Lothe confirmed his previous work which had been criticised because part of it was non-blind (Lothe *et al.*, 1982); the more recent trial confirms the benefit of Nutramigen in infant colic (Lothe and Lindberg, 1987). In the experience of these authors, infantile colic was related to cows' milk protein intolerance both in breast and formula fed infants. It seems quite amazing that a disorder which affects hundreds of thousands of babies is still lacking a proper trial in this country and that, with hundreds of professional workers running infant clinics, where there are thousands of screaming babies, we can only say that we *think* we believe in this or that as the cause. Many paediatricians do not regard cows' milk protein as of any importance in the aetiology of three-month colic.

The next example is failure to thrive, looking classically like coeliac disease. Typically, after a baby has been changed from breast milk to bottle feeding there is a catastrophic loss of weight and failure to thrive, but there is a dramatic recovery on a cows' milk-free diet. In the early 1970s we noted small fatty inclusions in the jejunal biopsy material, although the jejunal villi were quite well formed – and certainly not compatible with coeliac disease – an appearance now recognised as being characteristic of cows' milk protein intolerance.

Looking at the lower gastro-intestinal tract through a paediatric colonoscope, we can now visualise cows' milk haemorrhagic colitis, which is very similar to ulcerative colitis (Jenkins *et al.*, 1984). An expert colonoscopist can visualise the whole colon and the lower ileum as well. We can now reasonably say that most babies with colitis have cows' milk protein or

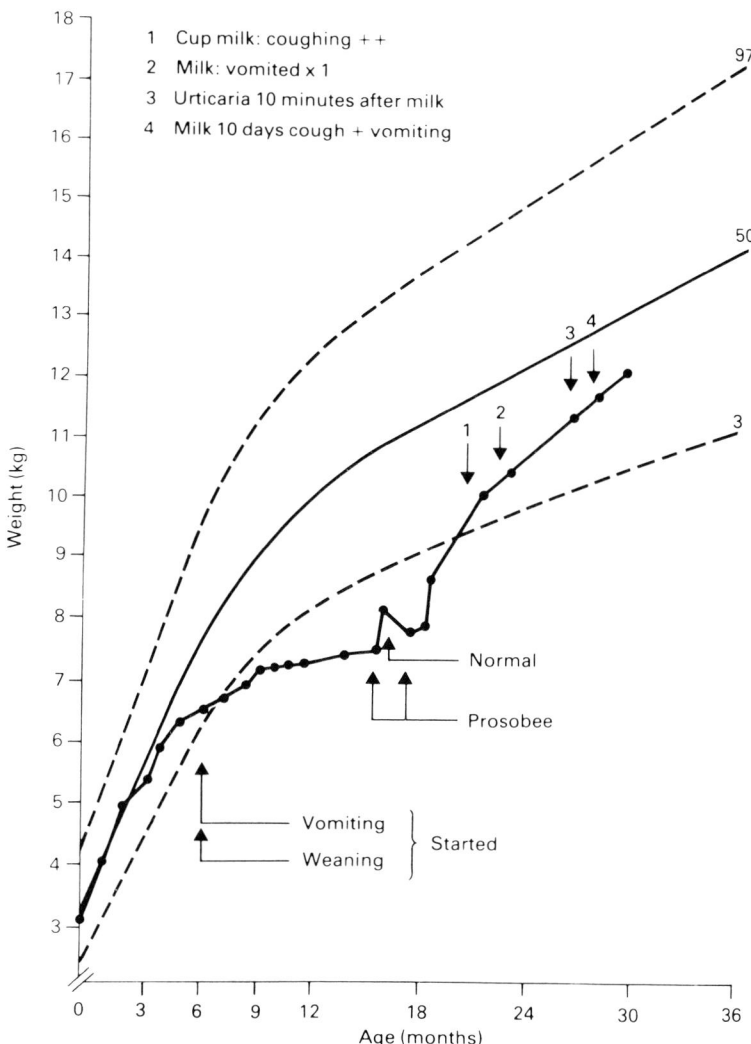

Figure 2   Effect of cows' milk with allergy on weight gain in an infant

multiple food intolerance until proved otherwise, but they should not be started on a soya formula because being immunologically stimulated they rapidly develop intolerance to soya protein also. It is quite important that these babies are fed with a protein hydrolysate formula such as Pregestimil. It is disappointing that we still have infants who have not been on a cows' milk-free diet referred for colonoscopy because of colitis-like symptoms.

Another common situation is that of a child who has no significant gastro-intestinal symptom but whose growth rate can be greatly improved by pre-scribing an elimination diet. The weight chart following this manoeuvre could be described as the 'drooping flower' type chart (Figure 2). For example, a baby after weaning started to lose weight. After starting her on a gluten-free, cows' milk-free diet she improved fairly rapidly. An initial jejunal biopsy was not done because of the urgency of the situation, but as the child recovered the biopsy showed normal intestinal mucosa. She was then challenged with gluten and her weight started to fall again but at the same time a second jejunal biopspy showed normal mucosa. This made it unlikely that she had coeliac disease. Gluten was then removed and she recovered; she was subsequently challenged with cows' milk and a further fall in weight occurred. Only when the diet was both cows' milk-free, gluten-free and egg-free did this child resume a normal growth pattern. At follow-up at the age of 7 years the child is thriving, growing along the 25th centile for weight, with absolutely no gastrointestinal symptoms and no positive tests to any food allergens. Nonetheless, I am convinced that this is an example of food intolerance, albeit transient.

The next example is of a severely allergic boy who is apparently allergic to nearly everything. Children such as this continue to give trouble and, as Dr Brueton pointed out, they switch over from their multiple food allergies and their eczema to respiratory and other problems as they get older. They are often rather slender, they itch all over and their weight chart, again, looks like a drooping flower, characteristic of food intolerance. The child I mentioned was put on a basic elimination or 'few foods diet' (for babies this normally consists of Nutramigen or Pregestimil and baby rice) and he did very well. When challenged with various foods his weight started to go down and so weight gain proceeded in a jagged manner. For this type of child to thrive all the therapeutic stops may have to be pulled out and all available therapeutic measures, including diet, medicines such as antihistamines, sodium cromoglycate, and steroid, both topical and systemic, may have to be used. Such treatment can be very difficult and some patients of this type are classed as having hyperimmunoglobulin E syndrome.

In the days before parenteral nutrition some of these children with severe symptoms including intractable diarrhoea simply wasted away and died. Twenty years ago cows' milk protein intolerance was rarely considered as a possible cause. We occasionally see the intractable diarrhoea syndrome, which frequently starts in babies who have had gastroenteritis and manifests as a continuation of diarrhoea without specific cause, for more than two weeks. Data on an interesting series of such infants, published by the Hospital for Sick Children, Great Ormond Street, show that of 82 infants 33% had coeliac disease and more than 10% cows' milk protein intolerance (Larcher et al., 1977). Another report, from Manchester, showed a response to breast milk (MacFarlane and Miller, 1984) and there are rare cases that are alleged to respond to the replacement of tap-water with purified or bottled mineral water. Originally such infants required parenteral feeding but our first manoeuvre nowadays is to put them onto Pregestimil and we now rarely see infants who need prolonged parenteral nutrition. It must be stressed that such infants require detailed investigations to exclude other causes for their diarrhoea, e.g., infections and other causes of failure to thrive.

Irritable bowel syndrome

This is a controversial topic, particularly amongst gastroenterologists treating adults, the majority of whom do not consider food intolerance as a likely cause of the condition with the exception of Dr Hunter and colleagues in Cambridge (Alun-Jones *et al.*, 1982). Having investigated many older children with chronic diarrhoea, I now put them on an elimination diet early in the course of investigation and am convinced that a proportion, perhaps 15–20%, have symptoms due to food intolerance. Julia, who is now about 18 years old, had lifelong abdominal pain and diarrhoea. Most investigations on her were negative and her condition was said to be emotional. When she was put on an elimination diet at the age of 12 years the diarrhoea stopped abruptly and she produced normal stools for the first time for years and her abdominal pain ceased. After the elimination diet she was challenged with one food after another and diarrhoea occurred only after potato. Dr Hunter and colleagues in Cambridge have found a number of different foods which worsen irritable bowel symptoms. It seems reasonable to give such patients a trial off the common food allergens for a period of two or three weeks as part of their routine investigation.

It is worth recalling at this point that before the role of gluten was discovered in coeliac disease this condition was often fatal. Today's patients with food intolerance can resemble those described with coeliac disease in the 1920s. The true incidence of coeliac disease, certainly as diagnosed by jejunal biopsy, seems to have diminished over the past decade in the Leeds area (Littlewood *et al.*, 1980), but the number of children recognised as having food intolerance has steadily increased (Minford *et al.*, 1982).

Laboratory tests

In my experience, investigations are not helpful except to rule out other disorders, e.g., jejunal biopsy to rule out coeliac disease. The main diagnostic weapon in this field is the elimination diet, a diet of few foods which excludes most of those likely to cause trouble. There are a number of different diets but it is better to take the advice of the local dietitian, who is familiar with her own particular version. Those who look for objectivity in medicine might like to refer to the paper by Wilson and colleagues (1982), who showed that in food-sensitive asthmatic patients pretreatment with the particular food could sensitise the patient, causing an enhanced bronchial reaction to histamine challenge without changing the resting peak expiratory flow rate. This is a demonstration of how the bronchi can be primed and sensitised by administration of a food.

Treatment of gastro-intestinal food allergy

Although dietary avoidance is the mainstay of treatment, some drugs are of value, e.g., antihistamines, ketotifen and corticosteroids.

Prognosis

Most infants become tolerant to food within three to four years. In our series of sixty-eight children, eighteen had recovered by the time we reviewed them, though some have continued with their food intolerance. Children with allergy to nuts seem to continue with this allergy and there are quite a number of older children whose symptoms have changed towards respiratory symptoms, especially those with a high IgE (Dannaeus and Inganas, 1981).

Prevention

Although breast feeding is promoted as a primary method of prevention, reported studies are contradictory (Burr, 1983). If one recommends exclusive breast feeding for four to six months, one should advise the mother regarding a sensible varied diet with no excess of any one particular food. Avoidance of inhalant allergens is also important – there is little point in excluding all the suspect dietary proteins and allowing the infant to roll about on the floor with the family cats and dogs! Dr Lingam has also mentioned the total allergen load and the need to look at every aspect of the patients' allergic problems. Our present practice in feeding infants who have shown allergy to cows' milk is to delay the introduction of allergenic foods (e.g., wheat, gluten, egg, fish) and leave their introduction until after the age of 9 months.

Summary of the problems

1. A lack of a specific test which can be readily applied in an ordinary clinic.

2. Double pathology. Food allergy needs to be thought of alongside other conditions.

3. The presence of allergens in breast milk, which many people still do not seem to have realised.

4. The acquisition of tolerance. A food that was giving trouble a month ago may not be giving trouble now but it does not mean it was not giving trouble earlier.

5. A variation on Meadow's Syndrome, or Munchhausen by proxy, in which mothers insist on their children having a restricted diet for which there is no justification.

6. Persisting professional ignorance which frequently fails to recognise the diagnosis, or does not recognise it at all.

REFERENCES

Alun-Jones, V., Shorthouse, M., McLaughlan, P., Workman, E. and Hunter, J. O. (1982). Food intolerance: a major factor in the pathogenesis of irritable bowel syndrome. *Lancet*, **ii**, 1115–17

Burr, M. L. (1983). Does infant feeding affect the risk of allergy? *Arch. Dis. Child.*, **58**, 561–5

Dannaeus, A. and Inganas, M. (1981). A follow up study of children with food allergy. Clinical course in relation to serum IgE- and IgG-antibody levels to milk, egg and fish. *Clin. Allergy,* **ii,** 533–9

Jakobsson, I. and Lindberg, T. (1983). Cow's milk proteins cause infantile colic in breast fed infants: a double blind crossover study. *Pediatrics,* **71,** 268–71

Jenkins, H. R., Pincott, J. R., Soothill, J. F., Milla, P. J. and Harries, J. T. (1984). Food Allergy: the major cause of infantile colitis. *Arch. Dis. Child.,* **59,** 326–9

Larcher, F., Shepherd, R., Francis, D. E. and Harries, J. T. (1977). Protracted diarrhoea in infancy. *Arch. Dis. Child.,* **52,** 597–605

Lessof, M. H., Wraith, D. G.., Merrett, T. G., Merrett, J. and Bruisseret, P. D. (1980). Food allergy and intolerance in 100 patients – local and systemic effects. *Quart. J. Med.* **49,** 259–71

Littlewood, J. M., Crollick, A. J. and Richards, I. D. G. (1980). Childhood coeliac disease is disappearing. *Lancet,* **ii,** 1359

Littlewood, J. M. and MacDonald, A. (1986). Clinical aspects of food allergy and intolerance. In Heatley, R. V., Losowsky, M. S. and Kelleher, J. (eds.) *Clinical Nutrition in Gastroenterology,* pp 202–33. Churchill Livingstone

Lothe, L., Lindberg, T. and Jakobsson, I. (1982). Cows' milk formula as a cause of infantile colic. A double-blind study. *Pediatrics,* **70,** 7–10

Lothe, L. and Lindberg, T. (1987). Cows' milk whey protein as a cause of infantile colic in formula fed infants. *Eur. Soc. Paediat. Gastroenterol. Nutr.* Lisbon

MacFarlane, P. I. and Miller, V. (1984). Human milk in the management of protracted diarrhoea of infancy. *Arch. Dis. Child.,* **59,** 260–5

Minford, A. M. B., MacDonald, A. and Littlewood, J. M. (1982). Food intolerance and food allergy in children: a review of 68 cases. *Arch. Dis. Child.,* **57,** 742–7

Walker-Smith, J., Harrison, J., Kilby, A., Phillips, A. and France, N. (1978). Cows' milk sensitive enteropathy. *Arch. Dis. Child.,* **53,** 375–80

Wilson, N. M. (1985). Food related asthma: a difference between two ethnic groups. *Arch. Dis. Child.,* **60,** 861–5

5

Oro-dental manifestations of food allergy

M. K. Basu

The mouth is the portal of entry of food and the site for its mastication. Consequently, the oral tissues come into contact with food stuff before it is propelled into the gastro-intestinal tract. In terms of food allergy, the mouth may be important as a possible site of sensitisation by a food allergen. Furthermore, in an already sensitised individual the mouth tissues may become the initial site of challenge, with symptoms of food allergy developing there.

The gastro-intestinal manifestations of food allergic disease include malabsorption of proteins, calcium and folic acid. All these are necessary for proper development and maintenance of the integrity of oro-dental tissues. It is not surprising, therefore, that oro-dental manifestations are to be found in patients suffering from food allergic disease, and quite frequently changes

Table 1 Symptoms and signs observed in seventy-nine children with cows' milk protein intolerance (from Buisseret, 1978)

Symptoms/signs	No. of patients	% of total
Flexural and perioral eczema	65	82
Asthma and/or rhinitis	74	93
Mismatch of height/weight centiles	46	58
Abdominal pain with constipation or diarrhoea	67	84

occur in the perioral tissues. In a study of the clinical features of seventy-nine children suffering from cows' milk protein intolerance Buisserett (1978) found perioral and flexural eczema in 82% of them (Table 1). Interestingly, the perioral eczema was provoked specifically by cows' milk protein. No other allergen would produce eczema in these children. The respiratory symptoms, on the other hand, could be provoked by commonly inhaled allergens such as pollen, house mites and animal dander.

Perioral eczema

This shows the typical clinical features of atopic dermatitis; that is, vesiculation of the skin at first, followed by weeping and crusting of the lesion around the mouth. It then develops into typical eczematous plaques on the skin of the cheeks and lips, and they are often itchy.

Under the microscope the surface epithelium shows intercellular oedema with vesiculation. The dermis is oedematous and contains neutrophils and plasma cells. There are variable numbers of eosinophils present as well. The eczematous lesions resolve on a cows' milk elimination diet and reappear when milk is added. The pathogenesis of perioral eczema in cows' milk protein allergy is not very clear. In some patients, at least, the histological picture, which resembles that of atopic dermatitis, suggests a local IgE-based reaginic reaction.

Intra-oral changes may occur in patients with food allergic disease. In a study of a hundred patients with food allergy Lessof and his colleagues (1980)

Table 2 Prominent symptoms in patients with food intolerance (from Lessof et al.)

	No. with each symptom	*Total no. of patients*
Group 1	Asthma 58	64*
	Eczema 37	
Group 2	Urticaria 18	22**
	Angioedema 8	
Group 3	Abdominal symptoms 11	14
	Rhinorrhoea 7	

*Twenty-three also had abdominal and nineteen had nasal symptoms. Seventeen had Group 2 symptoms, including lip swelling.
**Seven had abdominal symptoms, five had rhinorrhoea.

found eight with swelling of the lips due to angioedema (Table 2). In another study by Wraith and his colleagues (1979) twenty out of ninety-three patients (25%) were found to have swelling of the lips due to angioedema. A number of these patients also complained of mouth irritation – a burning sensation in the mouth with mild oedema. Many different foods were responsible for the symptoms which included lip swelling, and this was confirmed by putting the patients on elimination diets and provocation tests. During the provocation tests the lip swelling took about an hour to two hours to develop, suggesting an immediate IgE-based reaginic response to the allergen.

Angioedema

Angioedema may affect the whole of the lips or only a part of one lip. In some cases other oral tissues, such as the cheeks, tongue and submandibular tissues, can become oedematous and swollen. The lips become incompetent as a result of tongue enlargement and drooling of saliva occurs. The swollen tissues are soft and boggy to feel and they may be itchy and sensitive to touch. Microscopic examination of the lip mucosa shows pronounced oedema of the surface epithelium. There is much oedema in the lamina propria, which contains numerous neutrophils, a few plasma cells and quite a few eosinophils. With double staining techniques (immunoperoxidase/toluidine blue), the presence of numerous neutrophils, a few plasma cells and quite a few eosinophils. With double staining techniques (immunoperoxidase/toluidine blue), the presence of numerous IgE stained mast cells in the lamina propria can be demonstrated. This appearance is suggestive of reaginic hypersensitivity occurring within the lamina propria of the swollen oral tissues.

Oro-facial granulomatosis

Recently it has been realised that oro-facial granulomatosis – a disease in which non-caseating epithelioid granulomas form within the oral mucous membranes in the absence of any evidence of systemic granulomatous disease – can be a manifestation of food allergic disease. A 10-year-old child progressively developed swollen lips and cheeks over a period of one year. Fissures had developed on the swollen lips and these were deep and painful. The mucosa of the cheek became rough and cobble-stone-like in appearance. The swollen tissues of the lip and cheek were not soft and boggy but were firm and fibrous, causing movement of the lips and cheeks to become somewhat restricted.

Biopsies taken from the lip showed numerous non-caseating epithelioid cell granulomas to be present within the lamina propria and submucosa and also within the stroma of the lip muscles. The fibrous tissue in-between the granulomas showed features of non-specific chronic inflammation.

The patient was further investigated for underlying granulomatous disease but no evidence of Crohn's disease of the bowel or sarcoidosis or TB was found. The mouth lesions did not respond to treatment with mouth washes and local steroid application but they resolved when the patient was put on systemic prednisolone. However, remission was temporary and symptoms reappeared when prednisolone was stopped. It took two to three weeks for swelling of the lips to recur.

A recent publication (Patton et al., 1985) involved studying a group of fourteen patients with oro-facial granulomatosis who also complained of food or flavouring intolerance. A battery of patch tests was done on these patients and the results can be seen in Table 3. When put on elimination diets three patients showed complete remission of signs and symptoms while others showed partial remission. Our patient, described above, was also put on an oligo-allergenic diet and had remission of symptoms.

The pathogenesis of oro-facial granulomatosis is not clear. However, perivascular mononuclear cell infiltrates are found in the oral tissues, in addition to sarcoid granulomas. The mononuclear cells consist of lymphocytes and histiocytes. This microscopic picture and the fact that the oral lesions take days rather than hours to redevelop when the patients are taken off prednisolone suggest very strongly that delayed hypersensitivity mechanisms may be involved in the immunopathogenesis of oro-facial granulomatosis.

Table 3 Food flavouring intolerance in fourteen patients with oro-facial granulomatosis (from Patton et al, 1985)

Patient	Clinical	Patch test	Provoking factor	Response to withdrawal	Comment
CH	+	+ Cocoa	Dark chocolate	Partial	
JR	+	+ Cocoa	Dark chocolate	Partial	Crohn's
MB	+	+ Cinnamaldehyde	Vermouth, brandy, gin, toothpaste	Complete	Melkersson-Rosenthal
ME	+	Not done	Peanuts, cinnamon	Partial	
HM	+	+ Cinnamon	Curry	Partial	Melkersson-Rosenthal
JM	+	Not done	Wheat products, toothpaste	Complete	Urticarial rash with porridge
DM	+	Not done	Dairy products	Partial	Multiple allergies
AC	+	+ Cinnamaldehyde	Various toothpastes, tobacco products	Partial	Multiple allergies
CC	−	No reaction	Toothpaste	Partial	
SC	+	+ Cinnamon	Fruits and cinnamon	Partial	
LD	+	Not done	Wheat products, dairy products	Partial	Multiple allergies
GG	+	+ Cinnamon + Piperitone	Toothpaste	Partial	
LH	+	Not done	Wheat products, eggs	Complete	
CF	+	+ Carvone	Toothpaste	Partial	

Aphthous ulceration

This is a common disease and 10–20% of the population suffer from it. The ulcers occur in crops and are recurrent. They vary in shape, size, numbers and duration, and on the basis of these clinical features have been classified into major, minor and herpetiform types (Lehner, 1977).

Under the microscope the aphthous ulcers are similar and non-specific in that they all show evidence of ulceration of the surface epithelium, with a small lymphocyte predominant subacute inflammatory reaction in the lamina propria and submucosa initially. This later changes to a chronic inflammatory reaction, which is followed by healing.

The aetiology of aphthous ulceration is multifactorial and stress, infection by streptococcus sanguis, infection by herpesvirus hominis type 1, imbalance of sex hormones, and haematinic deficiency, which occurs in bout 30% of patients with aphthous ulceration, have all been suggested as aetiological factors.

We have studied a series of patients who presented with aphthous ulceration to determine any association between aphthous ulceration and systemic disease. We have found that between 4 and 6% of the patients have underlying coeliac disease, and that their aphthous ulcers heal and do not recur when they are put on a gluten-free diet (Asquith and Basu, 1978). In a series of a hundred consecutive patients presenting at the mouth ulcer clinic of our hospital, we found four coeliacs, six patients with Behcet's disease, eight with IgA deficiency, twelve with abnormal lactose tolerance and four with xylose malabsorption. In the other sixty-six patients we did not find any systemic abnormality.

Recently a study was conducted on nine patients who presented with severe aphthous ulceration of the mouth and who had normal jejunal biopsies with no evidence of villous atrophy (O'Mahoney *et al.*, 1985). Three of the nine patients showed raised serum anti-gliadin antibody levels and also increased numbers of intra-epithelial lymphocytes in the jejunal mucosal biopsies. Complete remission of aphthous ulceration occurred when the three patients were put on a gluten-free diet, and their levels of serum anti-gliadin antibodies returned to normal. Their mouth ulcers relapsed when they were challenged later with gluten, although their jejunal biopsies remained more or less normal in appearance. The other six patients did not show raised serum anti-gliadin antibodies and their ulcers did not respond to gluten-free diet. The results from this study and from our own studies suggest strongly that in some aphthous ulcer patients mouth ulceration may be a manifestation of gluten intolerance.

In order to study the relationship between aphthous ulceration and food allergy, we put thirty-two patients with aphthous ulceration on exclusion diets. The mouth ulcers responded to the exclusion diet in eleven cases: in seven to gluten withdrawal and in four to milk withdrawal. The mean number of ulcer-free days enjoyed after the patients had been on the elimination diet for four months was about three times more than the number of ulcer-free days enjoyed before they went on the diet.

These patients were challenged with the appropriate allergen by three different routes with a view to studying the mechanism of their mouth ulceration. We first challenged them, on two different occasions, through the oral route – that is to say, the patients only rinsed their mouths with the allergen, taking care not to swallow any of it. Seven of the eleven patients developed ulcers after this challenge, on both occasions.

On another occasion they were challenged via the stomach. The allergen was instilled directly into the stomach through a naso-gastric tube, thereby by-passing the mouth. Five of the eleven patients developed ulcers as a result.

The third time we used a combined route of challenge. Each patient was asked to swill the allergen around in his mouth and then swallow it, so as to make sure that it came into contact with both the mouth and the stomach tissues. Ten out of the eleven patients developed ulcers when challenged by this combined route.

From the results of this study we feel that in addition to Type 1 reaginic mechanisms, antigen-antibody mediated Type 111 hypersensitivity mechanisms may be important in the development of aphthous ulceration in food allergic disease. This hypothesis receives support from the microscopic appearance of the mouth ulcers. These show evidence of small vessel vasculitis in areas that are remote from the ulcer. The vessels also stain for IgG and complement C3 when stained by immuno-histochemical methods. This feature is not present in aphthous ulcers occurring in patients without systemic abnormalities.

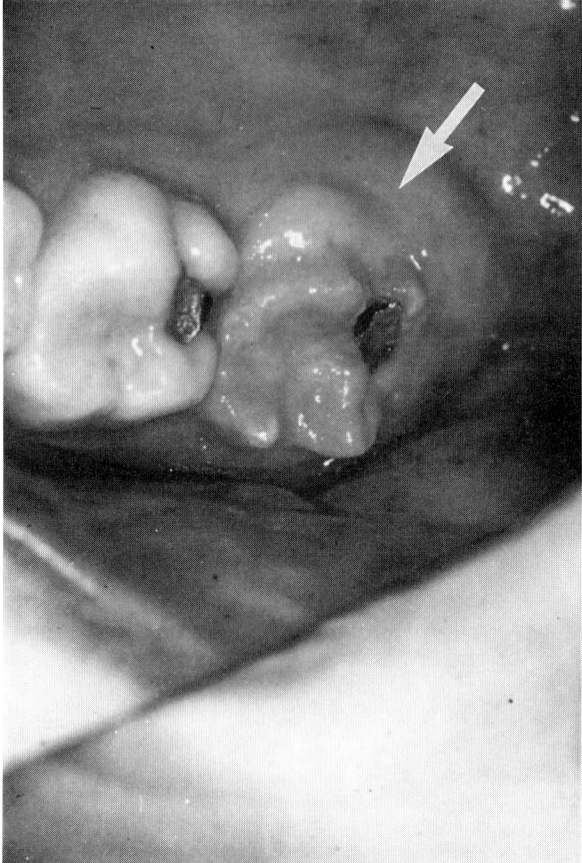

Figure 1 First permanent molar tooth in right maxilla showing signs of hypoplasia and hypomineralisation. Note that the deciduous molar tooth does not show such changes

Dental manifestations

Lastly, dental manifestations are sometimes found in children suffering from food allergic disease. The teeth show evidence of hypomineralisation and hypoplasia, as was found in the child shown in Figure 1 who suffered from coeliac disease. Presumably, the dental manifestations are caused by nutritional deficiency following malabsorption.

REFERENCES

Asquith, P. and Basu, M. K. (1978). Aphthous ulceration. In incidence of coeliac disease and gluten sensitivity. In McNicholl, B., McCarthy, C. E. and Fottrell, P.-F. (eds) *Perspectives in Coeliac Disease*. MTP Press, Lancaster

Buisseret, P. D. (1978). Common manifestations of cows' milk allergy in children. *Lancet*, **1**, 304–5

Lehner, T. (1977). Oral ulceration and Behcet's syndrome. *Gut*, **18**, 491–511

Lessof, N. H., Wraith, D. G., Merrett, T. G. Merrett, J. and Buisseret, P. D. (1980). Food allergy and intolerance in 100 patients – local and systemic effects. *Quart. J. Med.,* New series XLIX, No. 195, 259–71

O'Mahoney, C., O'Farrelly, C., Weir, D. G., Finch, T. and Feighery, C.F. (1985). Gluten sensitive oral ulceration in the absence of coeliac disease. *Br. Soc. Gastroenterol.,* Autumn meeting, 1985, abstract T5

Patton, D. W., Ferguson, M. M., Forsyth, A. and James, J. (1985). Oro facial granulomatosis: a possible allergic basis. *Br. J. Oral Maxillofacial Surg.,* **23,** 235–42

Sweatman, M. C., Tasker, R., Warner, J. O., Ferguson, M. M. and Mitchell, D. N. A. (1986). Oro-facial granulomatosis. Response to elemental diet and provocation by food additives. *Clin. Allergy,* **16,** 331–8

Wraith, D. G., Merrett, J., Roth, A., Yoman, L. and Merrett, T. G. (1979). Recognition of food-allergic patients and their allergens by the RAST technique and clinical investigation. *Clin. Allergy,* **9,** 25–36

6

Atopic eczema and other allergic disorders of the skin

A. J. Franklin and C. Blair

Atopic people form between one-sixth and one-third of the population, with up to 20% showing evidence of disease at some time in their lives. Of these, approximately half may have eczema for varying lengths of time and of varying severity. It is by far the commonest allergic disorder of the skin in children and represents a great deal of misery, discomfort and embarrassment to a lot of children and their parents, leading to sleepless nights, scratched and bleeding skin, infection, social withdrawal and emotional disturbance in many cases. Like the incidence of asthma, world-wide, the prevalence of eczema may be increasing.

Using Von Pirquet's definition of allergy as 'altered reactivity', it is possible to invoke the role of allergy in many skin diseases. Some inherited skin diseases such as ichthyosis may be associated with eczema in its autosomal dominant form, and the dry skin makes it more susceptible to irritants such as acids, alkalis and solvents. Virus-produced warts on the skin are common and most of these will disappear when the appropriate antibody is produced to eliminate the virus. Fungi are important because although they do not penetrate deeply into the skin they may produce chemicals which cause allergic inflammation and a generalised rash as also occurs in parasitic infestation, for example, scabies.

Urticaria is a more obvious allergic reaction, but it is not easy to find its cause. The intensely itchy 'nettle rash' or blister-like eruption and swelling which occurs on all areas of the body can appear and disappear within minutes or hours and there is often a time (related to exposure) factor which makes the diagnosis easy. Sometimes, however, fresh lesions may appear quickly so that the eruption seems to be continuous.

Some urticarias appear to be triggered by exposure to physical factors such as heat, cold, pressure, or exposure to water, irrespective of its temperature. These may also produce mediators similar to the allergic reactions. With foods the reaction can be an immediate and easily recognised Type I immune response (associated with the production of IgE) or delayed, possibly due to a Type III response, which is more difficult to identity from the history.

Urticaria is often self-limited, but deficiency of the enzyme C1 esterase inhibitor may cause excess oedema which could be life-threatening in certain sites, for example, on head and neck, and this can be corrected. The search for a causative food may be unrewarding as the condition usually responds fairly well to antihistamines and other drugs. Occasionally the reaction may be so severe as to produce a life-threatening swelling and obstruction in the mouth and larynx. Emergency administration of oral isoprenaline or subcutaneous or even intramuscular 1:1000 adrenaline solution may need to be given immediately and patients should be taught self-administration.

That foods should play a prominent role in the triggering of atopic eczema in young children seems probable, but it has proved very difficult to obtain satisfactory scientific proof. The time relationship referred to above is important and it should be possible to demonstrate that omitting foods from the child's diet leads to an improvement in the skin condition. Eczema is a chronic inflammatory disease of the subcutaneous layers of the skin as well as the

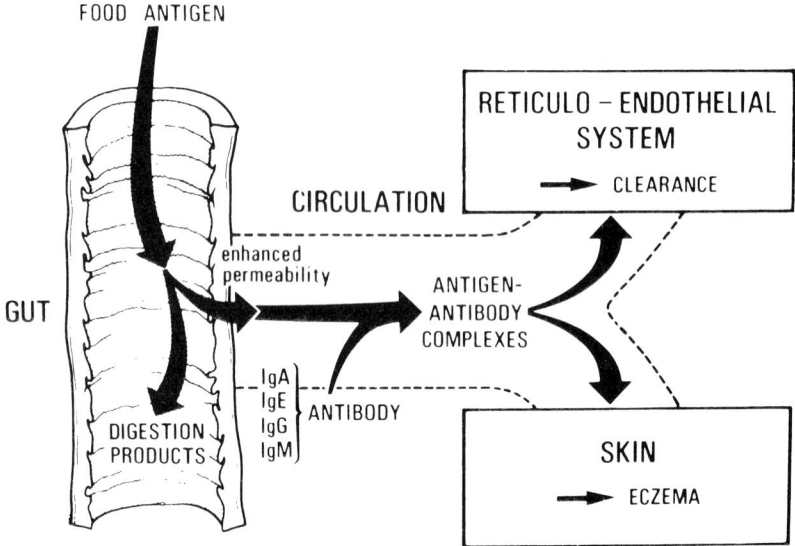

Figure 1 A hypothetical pathway for the pathogenesis of atopic eczema. In normal individuals food antigen-antibody complexes are formed in the circulation in small quantities after meals, and these appear to be rapidly cleared by the reticulo-endothelial system. The evidence suggests that such complexes are formed in greater quantities in individuals with atopic eczema, and that they have different properties. It seems possible that eczema results from their deposition in the cutaneous microvasculature

epidermis, so improvement (healing) may take several weeks. Once the inflammation has improved with an elimination diet it may then take several days to reappear after ingestion of the suspect food. The skin may be sensitive to other environmental factors – chemicals, for example, cosmetics and toilet preparations, or the house dust mite – so that challenges should be carried out in the patient's own home and not in hospital. Emotional factors can also play a part, making it difficult to obtain stable conditions in which to carry out a placebo-controlled double-blind trial. Such trials are not practical in ordinary clinical practice, but a simple elimination and challenge diet is worth while in any child whose eczema does not respond to simple emolient creams with or without hydrocortisone. Cases of mild eczema or with only small areas of skin involved hardly justify dieting, but continuing moderate eczema should be given a diet trial.

Atopic eczema is frequently a familial disease and it has been shown that elevated levels of IgE in the cord blood of the newborn infant precede and can predict the development of atopic disease subsequently. For a while the argument that breast feeding could prevent eczema was attractive, but this has not been proved and several studies have rather disproved it. Professor L. Businco showed that if atopic mothers exclusively breast fed their infants for six months or more, the incidence of eczema at one year was reduced, but such breast feeding had no effect on the non-atopic parents' children. Furthermore, mothers have described reactions in their infants after they themselves have consumed the suspect food (usually cows' milk; see Chapter 4). In the case of a breast fed infant, therefore, the mother needs to go on an elimination diet, as well as the infant.

A careful study by Atherton et al. in 1978 by means of a double-blind crossover trial excluding eggs and cows' milk showed that the skin definitely improved after exclusion of these foods and relapsed when they were reintroduced. A more recent study by Pike and Atherton (not yet published) has suggested that other foods could have a similar effect, although the results were less clear cut. The following foods were frequently implicated:

cows' milk
eggs
chicken and beef
artificial colourings and preservatives
citrus fruits.

Other foods less frequently caused skin inflammation in individual children subjected to elimination and challenge diets.

The method used by Pike and Atherton was to start the children on a simple empirical diet excluding the foods above (and any others suspected of causing reactions) for six weeks. At the same time environmental measures – controlling house dust, animals, humidity and home chemicals – were introduced. If there was no improvement after six weeks the diet was abandoned, but if the children improved the foods were then carefully challenged by reintroducing them one at a time at weekly intervals (even though some foods may take up to fourteen days before a reaction occurs), thus allowing identification and more prolonged exclusion of that food which caused a worsening of the eczema. Occasionally, in more resistant cases a full oligo-antigenic (few foods) diet or elemental diet is needed to identify the foods causing the skin reaction, but such diets put a lot of strain on families, are difficult to control, may lead to undernutrition and should always be supervised by an experienced dietitian. In the most severe cases or those which require the elimination of many common foods for long periods of time, the possibility of desensitisation should be considered (see Chapter 17). Supplements of calcium, zinc and vitamins may also be needed.

Most sufferers from eczema have very high IgE levels with multiple specific IgE RAST positive blood tests and often multiple positive prick skin tests. As in other systems where food allergy or intolerance may be the immediate cause of the condition, these tests do not correlate well with the causative foods. Some patients can have raised IgE levels and be clinically normal, whereas others can have normal tests and yet react on challenge to some foods. Until more accurate tests become available the diagnosis must rest on elimination and challenge diets as described elsewhere in this book. Difficult as these diets can be, the finding of a provoking food and its elimination from the diet can bring enormous relief to the chronic eczema sufferer and is usually well worth the effort involved. Subsequently, after an interval of approximately one to three years attempts may be made to reintroduce the excluded foods – especially if the patient is a young child, as it has been shown that tolerance tends to develop gradually, but not necessarily to all foods at the same rate, so that 90% of young children with eczema go into remission within five years.

As children grow older the importance of foods as a trigger factor for eczema may decline and be replaced by other allergies such as organic dusts and chemicals. At the same time foods sometimes trigger other target organs in the same person – for example, the lungs in asthma or the nose in chronic rhinitis – so that such children may not grow out of their food allergy altogether.

Conclusion

There is an allergic factor in many skin disorders; in atopic eczema, food is especially important. It is, however, only one of several factors and these should all be taken into consideration together when advising treatment.

REFERENCES

Atherton, D. J. (1982). Atopic eczema. *Clin. Immunol. Allergy*, **2** (1), 77–100

Businco, L. *et al.* (1983). Prevention of atopic disease in 'at risk' newborns' by prolonged breast feeding. *Ann. Allergy* **51 (2 Pt 2),** 296–9

Businco, L. *et al.* (1982). Result of a milk and/or egg free diet in children with atopic dermatitis. *Allergol. Immunopathol.* (Madr.) **10 (4),** 283–8

Hide, D. W. and Guyer, B. M. (1981). Clinical manifestations of allergy related to breast and cows' milk feeding. *Arch. Dis. Child.,* **56,** 172–5

Kjellman, N. I. M. and Johansson, S. G. O. (1976). IgE and atopic allergy in newborns etc. *Acta Paediat. Scand.,* **65,** 601–7

Matthews, D. J., Taylor, B., Norway, A. P., Turner, M. W. and Soothill, J. F. (1977). Prevention of eczema. *Lancet*, **i,** 321–4

O'Keefe, E. S. (1920). The relation of food to infantile eczema. *Boston Med. Surg. J.,* **183,** 569

Pike, M. G. and Atherton, D. J. (1985). Recent advances in the treatment of atopic eczema. *Prog. Child Health,* **2,** 13–28

Price, M. L. (1984) The role of diet in the management of atopic eczema. *Human Nutrition; Applied Nutrition,* **38a,** 409–15

Shacks, S. J. and Heiner D. C. (1982). Allergy to breast milk. *Clin. Immunol.* Allergy, **2** (1), 121–36

Taylor, B., Wadsworth, J., Wadsworth, M. and Peckham, C. (1984). Changes in the reported prevalence of childhood eczema since the 1939–45 war. *Lancet*, **ii,** 1255–7

Vickers, C. F. H. (1980). The natural history of atopic eczema. *Acta Dermatovenereol. (Stockholm)*, SUPPL. 92, 113–15

Warner, J. O. (1980). Food allergy in fully breast fed infants. *Clin. Allergy,* **10,** 133

7

Asthma and food allergy

D. G. Wraith

Asthma may be caused by allergy to foods as well as to inhalants. Inhalant allergies may be diagnosed from a knowledge of the environment, for example, animal pets, old bedding and dampness which would suggest house mite sensitivity, or a seasonal occurrence in the summer or late summer suggesting pollens or moulds, and these can be confirmed by skin prick tests. Foods as a cause of asthma have been very much overlooked. This is firstly because there is no obvious association between the foods and the symptoms, as the symptoms are caused by everyday foods which gradually build up and persist. Secondly, allergy skin (prick) tests and also IgE (RAST) tests are negative in the majority of these non-immediate symptoms, whereas in those with immediate symptoms, occurring soon after the food is taken, the reaction is obvious and the tests are usually positive. Food allergy was found to be a cause of asthma in a series of 170 patients aged under 15 years referred to an allergy and chest clinic in which I was involved. 62% of these also had inhalant allergies. There was a predominance of males (68%) in this group, compared with a predominance of females in a group of older patients whose asthma was caused by foods. In the absence of an obvious history or positive skin tests there were some features which were of help in the history, suggesting that food allergy might be a cause of symptoms, so that further investigations were carried out.

Features suggesting food allergy

(1) *Multiple symptoms.* The majority of these patients had other symptoms besides asthma, such as eczema, gastro-intestinal symptoms, behavioural problems and disturbance of micturition, which were also caused by food. Many also had ill-defined symptoms of tiredness, irritability and brain fag, which subsequently improved with food avoidance.

(2) *Family history.* Many had a family history of allergies in close relatives which suggested an allergic inherited basis.

(3) *Already known foods.* Some foods were already known to cause immediate symptoms which appeared soon after the food was taken and so were obvious.

This would suggest that there might be other hidden foods, and multiple foods were usually involved in food-related allergic disease.

(4) *Skin prick tests.* In those giving negative skin tests with inhalants, foods would be suspected; the majority had positive tests with inhalants as well as symptoms from foods, despite negative tests with the latter, so the possibility of symptoms from a combination of inhalants and foods should not be discounted, especially if there is not much improvement on excluding the inhalant allergens. Some of the positive tests with inhalants were not of significance because they were the results of previous sensitisation.

These features were of help in suggesting that food allergy might be a cause. However, it became increasingly obvious that food allergy was a much more frequent cause of asthma, and in combination with inhalants often caused more severe symptoms, so this should be considered as a possibility in all patients in whom avoidance of inhalants does not result in improvement.

Investigation of specific foods

In this series of patients under 15 years of age investigation of specific foods and additives was carried out mainly by elimination and reintroduction of foods. Stopping foods made the patient temporarily more sensitive, so a more definite reaction was obtained on their reintroduction, which would otherwise have been missed, as they were usually everyday foods. A small group of foods was stopped for ten days and then the foods restarted one at a time. The selection of foods for testing varied from patient to patient according to normal intake, including likes and cravings. Foods taken in larger amounts, or most frequently, were the chief culprits in producing asthma. Choice of foods was also influenced by ethnic habits or vegetarian preferences (more cereals and cheese in the latter), and in children artificial colouring taken in drinks and sweets was a major item. Selecting the foods for testing in this way was quicker and more efficient than by standardised diets which took much longer and missed essentials. Stopping and waiting for improvement would only result in confusion because many foods may be involved and some foods may be stopped unnecessarily. Regular peak flow measurements were very helpful as if there was a fall in the values foods could be stopped before more serious symptoms arose.

Precautions

Two extremely important precautions must be taken. (1) Take great care to avoid a severe reaction when reintroducing foods. Because the patient will be more sensitive after a brief abstinence, it is advisable to start by introducing a small quantity of foods and to increase the amount daily, stopping if peak flow readings rapidly fall or more general symptoms are produced. More sensitive patients may need to be admitted to hospital for challenge under medical supervision. (2) Adequate nutrition must be preserved, especially if the patient has previously been on a restricted diet. Supplements of vitamins, minerals or elemental food mixtures may be necessary. Suitable alternative foods may be substituted for some items.

Confirmation

If there is any doubt about a food, confirmation may be necessary by subsequent rechallenges. Occasionally foods taken by mistake will provide this; for example, sweets with colouring or medicines with colouring may be taken and increase the symptoms. In very busy clinics it is not normally possible to carry out blind tests and to disguise foods, sometimes in large quantities for several days.

Foods and symptoms

Table 1 shows the main food materials which caused asthma in this series of patients under 15 years of age.

Table 1   170 patients under 15 years of age with food allergy

Main foods, etc.	Number of patients
Milk	94
Colouring	71
Egg	62
Wheat	13
Cheese	11
Preservatives	10
Others	30

A few patients were affected by one food only but in several patients many foods were involved. Colourings and preservatives occur in many foods, sweets and drinks, and also in many tablets and medicines. Many patients with wheat sensitivity were also sensitive to other cereals, for example, corn, oats and rye, although rice is usually tolerated. Small amounts of corn starch may be found in tablets.

The item 'Others' in Table 1 included yeast, coffee, nuts, tomatoes, pork, fish and citrus fruits.

Comparison with patients over the age of 15 years shows that there was a much wider range of foods causing asthma in the older group. In the younger group the main foods responsible were milk, food colouring and egg. Table 2 shows the foods responsible in the older group.

Table 2   150 patients over the age of 15 with food allergy

Main foods, etc.	Numbers of patients
Milk	71
Wheat and other cereals	65
Egg	30
Cheese	25
Yeast	22
Colouring	25
Preservatives	16
Others	57

The majority of these patients had a similar range of other allergic symptoms to those found in the younger group. However, the frequency of the symptoms differed, with more arthralgia and lethargy and mood changes rather than hyperactivity. The above figures would suggest that allergies to foods depend on the relative amounts which are habitually taken. Avoidance of excess amounts of foods, especially artificial colouring in those with an allergic background, as suggested by family history or known allergies, would therefore help to prevent the development of allergies. Cravings for foods such as chocolate are often a cause of allergy, and artificial colouring is one of the largest causes of psychological and urticarial symptoms.

Examples

(1) A boy aged 7 had severe asthma in the summer. Skin prick tests showed a positive reaction for grass pollen, but desensitisation to pollen did not help very much. Stopping drinks of orange squash, of which he had more in the summer, resulted in cessation of his asthma.

(2) Morning peak flow levels for a boy aged 9 with a long history of asthma rose within twenty-four hours after certain foods were removed from his diet (see Figure 1). On reintroduction of these foods, values fell over three to four days, thus indicating the dramatic improvement from dietary control in asthmatic patients with a low tolerance to preservatives and colourings.

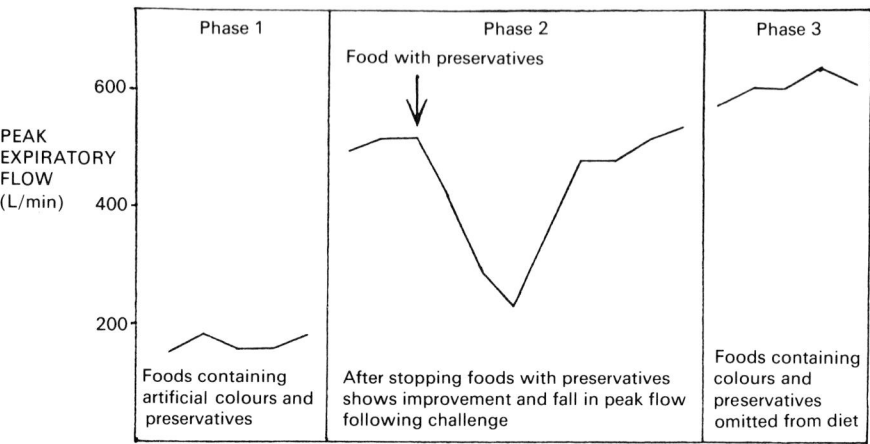

Figure 1 Effect of food additives on asthma

(3) A 40-year-old male had morning and evening peak flow breathing tests and kept a diary of all foods, etc. eaten. He showed improved values when pork, ham and bacon were omitted from his diet. Several other allergeric foods were found later and all were confirmed by a fall in peak flow values on their reintroduction (see Figure 2).

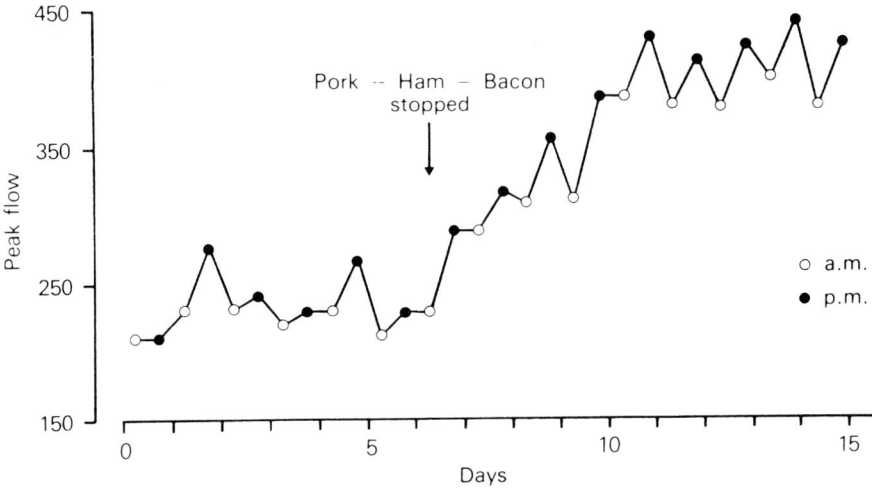

Figure 2   Effect of pork products on an asthmatic male adult

Other symptoms caused by foods

An association of other symptoms with asthma would also suggest food allergy. The majority of patients in this series did have other symptoms and they were often multiple (see Table 3).

Table 3   128 patients under 15 years with allergic symptoms in addition to asthma

Symptom	Number of patients
Eczema	59
Gastro-intestinal symptoms (mainly diarrhoea, abdominal pain or both)	26
Psychological symptoms (mainly hyperactivity)	21
Rhinitis	17
Urticaria	11
Enuresis	10
Joint symptoms	5

Many, in addition, had lesser degrees of irritability, tiredness, and poor sleeping patterns. All these symptoms were found to be caused by foods or additives and were relieved when the foods which were often similar to those causing asthma were stopped, though different foods may cause different symptoms.

Management

Many of these patients had severe asthma but food allergy had been over-looked. Treatment with continuous inhalers and recurrent courses of oral steroids were frequently able to be withdrawn once the offending foods had been discontinued. Those very sensitive to particular foods needed to stop them completely, though this was sometimes difficult in children because of school meals or food and sweets offered by friends. Artificial colouring in medicines was also an important cause in some patients. It is important to ensure that nutrition is adequate at all times, so consultation with a dietitian is essential. Many patients require supplementary vitamins and minerals. Oral sodium cromoglycate (Nalcrom) was very helpful in many of our patients as this enabled small amounts of foods to be taken which otherwise could not have been.

Conclusions

1. Food allergy is a very important cause of asthma but is easily overlooked. Greater awareness of this is necessary.
2. The immediate history and skin prick tests are often not helpful, but some features which suggest the possibility of food allergy have been given.
3. Maintenance of adequate nutrition is very important.

8

Hyperactivity – an allergic disorder?

A. J. Franklin

Innumerable small children appear to become overactive physically, disobedient, intolerant of frustration, aggressive (kick, bite and hit parents and other children), scream, rush about, throw things, seem miserable, will not sleep, cannot settle to learn or perform any other constructive activity after a regular diet of squashes, sweets, flavoured crisps, beefburgers and other foods with quantities of colouring, sugar and other additives. Some of these children appear to be so sensitive that they react to common staple foods, but not usually if they are grown organically. This suggests that agricultural chemicals may be incorporated into growing plants and battery-reared animals in sufficient amounts as to affect sensitive children and adults.

Many parents believe that the way that their children behave may have something to do with food allergy and they take them to clinics, demanding some kind of allergy tests to find out about it. One can sympathise with the parents of these impossible, awkward children who are quite difficult to manage in a surgery; to have to live with them twenty-four hours a day for seven days a week is quite daunting. It is generally agreed that hyperactivity is more common in boys and 'Fidgety Phil who couldn't sit still' is by no means a modern character. It was the German physician Heinrich Hoffmann who characterised him in his children's poem. At meal-times he would fidget about, push the table over, pull the cloth off the table and land everything on the floor to the great distress of his parents, so in fact, although he may seem to be a modern character, Fidgety Phil has been with us a long time.

The paediatrician Frederick Still commented on the condition in an article in *Lancet* in 1902, and two famous Englishmen were regarded as hyperactive at the beginning of this century, Winston Churchill and Thomas Edison, who was regarded as ineducable in his day. In the 1930s came the observation that, although actually a stimulant, the drug benzedrine switched off the hyperactive behaviour of some of these children and made them more educable (Bradley, 1937). From that observation came the tremendous surge in the 1960s, in the USA particularly, of treating these children with drugs, which brought a backlash in the present decade away from drugs altogether. In the 1970s the late Dr Ben Feingold surprised the world by suggesting that hyperactivity might be due to chemicals in the diet. In fact, it was interesting that Ben Feingold himself did not regard hyperactivity as an allergic disorder but he noticed that when he gave aspirin-sensitive children a salicylate-free diet some of them stopped being hyperactive. He was working on aspirin allergy at the time.

What is hyperactivity?

Hyperactivity is a chronic, pervasive deficiency in attention span and impulse control, and overactivity (Table 1). It describes the child who stands out from the rest, not just a child whose behaviour is at the end of a normal spectrum,

Table 1 Summary of the Hyperactive Child Syndrome

1 The term 'Hyperactive Child Syndrome' should be used to denote a behavioural syndrome only, with no implication as to aetiology.
2 The syndrome is more common in boys, begins early in life and is characterised by four cardinal symptoms: hyperactivity, impulsivity, distractibility and excitability.
3 Antisocial behaviour, specific learning disabilities and depressive symptoms occur in many, but not all, children with the syndrome.
4 Children with this syndrome form a heterogeneous group. It is likely that many aetiologic factors either alone, or in combination, can lead to the syndrome.
5 Epidemiological studies indicate that the syndrome is relatively common in the general population and a leading cause of referral to child guidance clinics

From Cantwell, D. P., 1975.

though of course there are degrees of disturbed behaviour. Hyperactive children are distinguished by their degree of motor restlessness, their fidgetiness, their 'squirminess', as it has been described in some places. They are very impulsive children, they do not stop and think, they will quite happily jump out of windows, or rush across main roads, quite oblivious to danger. Emotional immaturity is one very obvious feature of these children. They seem to be for ever being grumbled at by their parents and told to 'grow up'. A refusal to conform alternates with being overdependent upon their parents, and they lack confidence. At the other end of the scale they will suddenly react very strongly and become extremely aggressive to other children, to other adults, to anybody around, particularly anyone who tries to confine or frustrate them. They cannot tolerate discipline, and in a classroom situation they seem to be abnormally sensitive to incoming stimuli, so that almost anything can distract them from what they are doing onto the next thing, which makes them non-achievers and undermines their self-confidence.

This condition has been found in association with established medical conditions such as epilepsy and mental handicap but I wish to separate the condition here from those particular associations. Another association is with delayed language development and deafness. A particular interest of mine has been a relationship to sleep disorders. I was very impressed by the number of babies who would not sleep but who screamed perpetually during the first few months of life, and Doris Rapp (Chapter 10) describes the baby *in utero* being rather vicious. These children just do not sleep and when they cannot sleep they seem to lie awake and scream for hours.

The brain damage and hyperactivity story relates to studies which were done in asphyxiated infants where it was noticed that toxic damage could give rise to hyperactivity, and of course a number of the learning problems

Table 2   Results of pre-natal hypoxia

Asphyxia at or before birth selectively damaged the brain stem.
Maximal damage occurred to rapidly growing areas.
Further damage results from haemorrhage, contusions, drugs and brain compression.
Slight hypoxic damage→sleep and feeding problems.
Severe hypoxic damage→hypotonia, apathy and abnormal EEG.
Posterior brain ischaemia→visuo-spatial, verbal and learning problems.
Thymic damage→hyperactivity and attention deficit disorders.

Table 3   Long-term follow-up of asphyxiated infants

Three out of eight infants had behavioural disturbances: bad temper, excess backchat, excess rage, excess stubbornness.
Three out of eight infants had motor abnormalities with hyperactivity.
Diffuse damage usually produced hyperactivity under 3 years of age.

From Brown, J. K., 1976

are associated with it (Table 2). In Brown's study of a small group of asphyxiated infants which he followed up (Table 3) he found that three out of eight of them had behavioural disturbances which are the ones which most parents are very aware of: excessive rage, excessive backchat and excessive stubbornness, and three out of eight had a motor abnormality as well. However, brain damage probably accounts for less than 5% of hyperactive children.

To answer the question, 'Is this truly a medical disorder or are we dealing with a purely behavioural syndrome' – because it has been traditionally the province of the child guidance clinic and the psychologist to deal with this in the past – we set up a small study to investigate the possible allergic and other associations.

Study protocol

Children were selected mainly by Health Visitors on purely clinical criteria. Those who had had previous child guidance, psychiatric treatment, epilepsy or other neurological abnormalities were excluded, and admission to the study depended on scoring 17 or more on Connors' Parent Symptom Questionnaire*. The resulting highly selected group of thirty children aged between 3 and 13 years had a primary psychosocial behavioural disorder.

A questionnaire was sent to the parents, asking about their own health, their background, where they lived, environmental pollution, pregnancy and birth history of the children, to see if there were any genetic or environmental factors in the families themselves that might give rise to the children's disorders. Within the limitations of a district hospital simple tests were carried

* Details of this questionnaire can be found in Barkley's *Hyperactive Children* and Rapp's *Allergies and the Hyperactive Child*.

Table 4   Investigations

Skull X-ray
EEG
RAST screen – four inhalants – three foods
Hair mineral analysis
Food exclusion and challenge

out (Table 4), but not all the children completed all of the tests. Some had audiograms and immunological profiles; all had a RAST screen for allergy to common foods and common inhalants and a hair analysis for minerals, looking particularly for evidence of possible lead poisoning. Some had urine concentration tests, because one of the symptoms that emerged very early on was an excessive thirst, but they certainly were not diabetic.

All children were started on an exclusion and challenge diet under the supervision of a dietitian. It was not possible to have a controlled group because parents had spread the word and they all turned up having started on some kind of diet, so that a control diet had to be abandoned. The main variable was whether or not they had professional psychological guidance for six months; at the end of the six months a crossover was arranged. Psychological tests were conducted by our educational psychologist colleagues in the child guidance clinic, using the appropriate WISC subtests.

Information from the parents' questionnaire

The family

Surprisingly, considering the divorce figures in this country, the majority of the children in the study seemed to come from settled homes. Many of the mothers did not go out to work. The children were not necessarily first children with inexperienced parents, but were sometimes the second or third. They were not only children, they often had siblings and we were particularly impressed by the sort of illnesses which the parents also admitted to. These were mainly of the atopic variety (Tables 5 and 6).

Table 5   Family structure – thirty families

28 stable marriages; 2 divorced single parents
children: 13 firstborn, 12 second, 4 third
9 children had 2 siblings, 16 had 1, 5 were the only child

Table 6   Associated illnesses in parents

Migraine	17	Eczema	8
Asthma	14	Hay fever	5
Catarrh	13	Other allergy	10

Pregnancy

Twenty-four of the thirty mothers had a normal pregnancy and even the abnormal ones were not particularly outstanding for their abnormality. About one-third had hyperemesis and a minority smoked. About half of them described the baby as very active and only four as not very active (Table

Table 7 Pregnancy features – thirty families

24 normal; 6 complicated
 9 hyperemesis
28 gained weight, 2 lost weight
23 did not smoke, 2 smoked more than 15 cigarettes per day
13 took extra vitamins
Baby active *in utero*: very active 15, moderately active 11, not very active 4
Type of delivery: Normal 26, forceps 1, LSCS 3

7). There was nothing significant about the type of delivery, and birth weights ranged from 2.5 to 4.8 kg. The majority (eighteen) of the children were breast fed but thirteen had early feeding problems. Three seemed to have delay in speech development and the male/female ratio was 14:1, which is fairly characteristic of this syndrome. Two were adopted.

Problems in the children (Table 8)

Many of the children had upper respiratory problems. Of the behavioural symptoms which were admitted to, restlessness came out top but abnormal thirst was high on the list also. Table 9 shows when hyperactivity was first noticed. In a third of the children the parents were already complaining before the baby was 1 year old, so the syndrome develops early in infancy, only in very few cases does it begin after the age of 5 years. The older children who were seen in the study produced their first symptoms in the preschool years. Twenty-eight children came from homes that were heated by gas, which could be a factor, as has been mentioned elsewhere (Rapp, 1979, and see Chapter 10).

Test results

The X-rays were all normal. Although about one-fifth of the children had minor abnormalities on the EEG the neurophysiologist could not say what he thought these abnormalities were due to. Perhaps they have some problem here in that they are not used to looking at EEGs on normal children, or allegedly normal children who are not referred with neurological problems, so one was not sure whether this was a normal finding or not. Considering the immunoglobulins, one child had a T-cell deficit, three had opsonisation defects and eight had a raised total IgE. Looking at the specific IgEs, to our great surprise we found not a single child who gave a positive RAST to food; the positive ones were to inhalants. The hair mineral analyses were very confusing. High levels of copper and lead had been implicated in hyperactivity; in our study the copper levels were normal and the lead levels not

Table 8 Problems in the children

Behavioural

Restlessness	27	Fits/tantrums	20
Abnormal thirst	25	Impulsive	20
Crying/screaming	23	Aggressive	15
Poor concentration	22	Clumsy	13
Sleep problems	22	Poor appetite	13

Physical

Catarrh and ear infections	15	Diarrhoea	6
Chest infections	15	Adenoidectomy and Grommets	3
Eczema	14	Tonsillectomy	2
Abdominal colic	9	Broncho-pneumonia	1
Deafness	8	Hernia	1
Vomiting	7		

Table 9 First noticed overactivity

From birth	10
1–1$\frac{1}{2}$ years	9
2 years	7
3 years	3
5 years	1

particularly high. Obviously one should not have lead in one's blood but most urban children do have and we tested the hair of a few non-hyperactive children for comparison and the results were almost the same. Mineral deficiencies, especially of zinc, magnesium and manganese, may be worth correcting but there was no convincing diagnostic pattern. One interesting child had a very high mercury level. She had swallowed the end of a mercury thermometer two years previously and this was still reflected in her hair.

Figure 1 shows the Connors' scores, which fell in every case in the first six months. There could have been strong placebo effect with dieting and one might expect that to happen. As they were followed through for eighteen months, although some of them went up again, the majority seemed to go on down and in the third phase, when Evening Primrose Oil was introduced, the scatter went in all directions. At the end of the trial the scores on the right-hand side of the chart were generally lower than the scores at the beginning, and this was attributed mainly to dieting.

Diet challenge

The initial diet excluded dairy foods, food additives, food colouring, wheat, milk and tap water. After two weeks foods and additives were introduced weekly until they arrived at a diet which the parents thought was satisfactory, positive-reacting foods having been excluded. This diet was continued for six months. The children were reviewed after two and six months, when a reassessment was made using the Connors' score. Fifteen of the children were

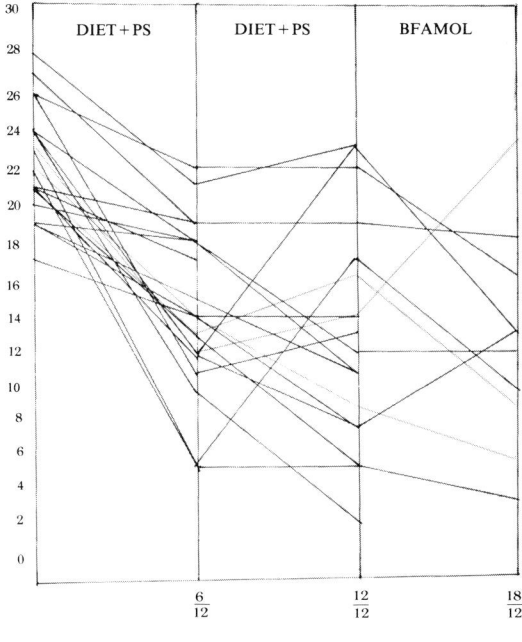

PROGRESSIVE CONNORS RATING SCORES

Figure 1 Changes in Connors Scores over an eighteen month period.

seen by the educational psychologist, who arranged group therapy for parents and children, three or four times in the six months' period. At the end of six months the groups switched over and we tried to see whether there was an effect from psychological counselling separate from the diet. This was done by looking at the IQ scores. Although very few children actually completed this (because of logistic difficulties), it was difficult to show any effect on the children from the psychological counselling, but the parents did gain confidence. One child bumped up his IQ score more than 20 points and it went on rising, which made tremendous difference to his school performance. A few did not respond at all and five showed a fall in Connors' score in the first six months, but crept up again in the next six months. That particular sequence was with psychological counselling first and diet alone second. When these were done the other way round there seemed to be rather bigger effects from the diet – some of which were cancelled out later – but not many of these were very significant.

The foods that seemed to be the most troublesome were the food colourings and the food flavours (Table 10), but chocolate is quite high up on the list and also cows' milk and tap-water (see Appendix 1). Tap-water in this country is certainly not pure water and something like 3500 additives have been recovered from it.

These findings may be compared with a rather more careful trial carried

Table 10   Food causing hyperactive behaviour

Azo-dyes and flavours	25
Tap-water	12
Chocolate	9
Cows' milk	7
Wheat	5
Apple	4
White bread, sugar, cheese	3
Ice-cream, banana, oranges, egg, tomato	2 each
Coffee, yoghurt, monosodium glutamate	1 each

out at the Hospital for Sick Children at Great Ormond Street by Egger, Soothill and colleagues in conjunction with the Institute of Psychiatry. They selected seventy-six children who were admitted to the trials by clinical observation and on completing a Connors' scale, but all of them were considered to be socially handicapped because of their condition. Thirty-seven of these children, based on Rutter's definition, were in families with adverse psychosocial conditions. Thirty were atopic on prick testing to five or more antigens, but not specifically to foods. About half of these were in the adverse psychosocial conditions group. A majority of the children had abdominal symptoms, quite a lot had headaches, aching limbs, chronic rhinitis, skin rashes and mouth ulcers, but the most exciting thing which came out of this study was that fourteen of the children had fits which responded to dietary treatment. A further trial has been undertaken to explore this aspect. In their study design they put all the children on an oligo-antigenic diet, as I had done, with supplementary calcium and vitamins. After reintroduction of the foods, the ones that caused the symptoms were selected for a double-blind trial in two groups on a crossover basis. Twenty-eight children completed this part of the trial. Symptoms returned much more frequently on the active than on the placebo material.

Their results were not dissimilar. Sixty-two children improved on the oligo-antigenic diet, and twenty-one of them achieved normal behaviour. Of the fourteen who had fits, thirteen became fit-free and that was really a most startling finding. As one perhaps might expect, the dietary response was less marked where there were adverse psychosocial factors, because they were not actually dealing with the psychosocial problems at this time. Only 50% of the children were atopic, but it is worth noting that 71% of the children exposed to adverse psychosocial factors, such as family mental disturbance, inconsistent parental control, lack of emotional warmth from caring adults or success at school, benefited from the dietary manipulation. In most the Connors' scores showed a marked drop from active to placebo. There are a few that obviously did not respond to the diet and it did not really matter which order they were in, except that those on placebo first were given higher scores by their parents than when assessed in reverse order. The placebo was a sort of lentil soup which was found to be non-reactive in the children. Forty-eight foods were incriminated, artificial colourants and preservatives being the commonest provoking substances, but *no child was sensitive to these alone*. Chocolate is very high on their list and this may be an important reason why some other trials using chocolate as placebo failed to show much effect from adding azo-dyes. There is practically no food there that one could say was totally safe except those that most young children will not eat – cabbage, lettuce, cauliflower, celery, goat cheese and duck eggs. It is worth re-emphasising that the children did not react only to additives but they also reacted to other foods and there did not seem to be a correlation between the food additives, the food colours and salicylate-containing foods. Keith Connors concluded after several trials that less than 5% of children who are genuinely hyperactive have some specific sensitivity to the artificial colours.

The answer to the question, 'Is hyperactivity an allergic condition?' is probably negative but allergy may indeed contribute to hyperactivity. The condition should probably be regarded as multifactorial. The genetic factor may well operate as it does in atopic children. Birth injury may have something to do with it in a few cases. The parental management of the child undoubtedly has to be looked at; for example, the child who is persistently allowed to run wild undoubtedly is going to go on behaving like that. Though behaviour modification does come into the management of such children, it will be no good trying to manage a child who is being driven mad by some of the things to which he is being exposed by eating, smelling or living with them, unless some attempt is made to find and exclude them first.

Conclusion

'Hyperactivity' is a term that should be used to denote a behavioural syndrome without necessarily implying an aetiology. There are four cardinal symptoms: hyperactivity, impulsivity, distractibility, and excitability associated with antisocial behaviour and learning difficulties. Hyperactive children form a heterogeneous group but that means that aetiological factors need to be looked at in some depth. It is not sufficient, if a child walks into your consulting room and starts to throw everything around and jump all over the place, to assume that either he is allergic to milk or he has bad parents. There is more to it than that and it requires time and effort to sort out. Dr Menzies (Chapter 11) believes that numbers of such children are not diminishing, despite a great deal of psychological research and a falling birth-rate, so that an environmental approach seems well justified before referring on to the child guidance clinic for behavioural modification.

REFERENCES

Barkley, R. A. (1982). *Hyperactive Children: A Handbook for Diagnosis and Treatment*. Wylie and Sons Ltd

Bradley, C. (1937). The behaviour of children receiving benzedrine. *Am. J. Psychiat.*, **94**, 577–585

Brown, J. K. (1976). *Recent Advances in Paediatrics*, Vol. V, pp 57–82. Churchill Livingstone, Edinburgh

Cantwell, D. P. (1975). *The Hyperactive Child*. Spectrum, New York

Connors, C. K. (1980). *Food Additives and Hyperactive Children*. Plenum Press, New York and London

Egger, J. *et al.* (1985). Controlled trial of oligo-antigenic treatment in the hyperkynetic syndrome. *Lancet*, 9 March, 540–5

Feingold, B. (1975). *Why Your Child is Hyperactive.* Random House, New York

Rapp, D. J. (1979) *Allergies and the Hyperactive Child*, pp 69 and 188. Sovereign Books, New York

Rutter, M. L. *et al.* (1975). *A Guide to a Multi-axial Classification Scheme for Psychiatric Disorders in Childhood and Adolescence.* Institute of Psychiatry, London

Schrag, P. and Divoky, D. *The Myth of the Hyperactive Child and Other Means of Child Control*

Still, G. F. (1902). The Goulstonian Lectures on some abnormal psychical conditions in children. *Lancet*, **1**, 1008–1012; 1077–1082; 1163–1168

9

Food additive sensitivity – a clinical trial

G. Supramaniam

Food additive sensitivity is a frequently recognised clinical problem. Many parents have reported symptoms which started after introducing a specific food. The symptoms and signs attributable to adverse reactions to foods include acute shock-like reactions, chronic gastro-intestinal manifestations such as vomiting, abdominal pain, diarrhoea, malabsorption and enteropathy, and occasionally respiratory manifestations such as rhinitis, cough and wheezing. The commonest manifestation one sees with food additives is urticarial rashes and eruptions. Rash in eczema may be aggravated in some patients and in others urticarial rashes may be the presenting symptom. There are central nervous system manifestations such as headache, apathy, irritability, moodiness and, as mentioned in Chapter 8, behaviour changes and hyperactivity.

Examples

A child who had a dry skin had a mild skin eruption which got worse after the child was given a fizzy drink, and which lasted for about forty-eight hours. The mother could identify the rash as coming on after giving the drink.

A 13-month-old child first presented with a history of not gaining weight. The child was born at term by normal delivery and there were no neonatal problems. Neither were there any problems at the time of introduction of solid food. Subsequently, when the child was about 14 months old the mother started introducing convenience foods, and at that stage she noticed that the child was vomiting and there was a behaviour change. She immediately stopped giving the child what is called 'convenience' food, whereupon the child started losing weight. She was admitted to hospital and various investigations were done, including a jejunal biopsy, but no abnormality was found. At that stage the child was put onto a normal diet and although the mother initially disagreed, after some persuasion she allowed us to do this and continued with it at home. Four months later the child was obviously thriving when seen in the clinic.

The trial

We decided to look at a specific group of children who presented with angioedema and urticaria. The symptoms can either be transient or persistent. The transient ones, which may be associated with viral infections or bacterial infections caused by beta-haemolytic streptococci or even gastro-intestinal infection caused by Giardia, may respond to treatment with antihistamines or treatment of the underlying infection. In the persistent group there may be a subgroup with an easily identifiable cause and in such instances avoidance measures may help, but these patients may also require antihistamines on some occasions. In another subgroup of patients there may be no identifiable cause and when commenced on a colouring and preservative free diet, a significant improvement may be observed; others show no improvement. Patients who showed significant improvement were admitted for a double-blind formal challenge. There were forty-three patients in this group, whose

Table 1   Presenting symptoms in the forty-three children in the study

Urticaria and pruritis	43
Angioedema	32
Rhinitis	17
Wheezing	4
Swollen lower eyelids	3
Diarrhoea	2
Recurrent	2
Behavioural disturbances	3

presenting symptoms were as shown in Table 1. All these children had multiple symptoms. There were twenty-one males and twenty-two females, with an age range between 3 years and 4 months and 14 years. The symptom frequency varied between one attack every three months to one attack every two weeks, the mean being one attack every two months. The duration of the reactions lasted from one day to one week and the duration of the problem in these forty-three patients was from eight weeks to six months.

Some of the parents were able to identify the precipitating factors – commonly fizzy drinks, milk, cheese, chocolate, orange drinks, fish and fish fingers, tomatoes, blackberries and strawberries – but in a large proportion of cases the cause was not known.

After a detailed history taking and examination the children were put on a colouring, preservative and salicylate-free diet by a dietitian who recommended the diet and saw them regularly before they came back to the clinic in the second week. All the children improved significantly while they were on the diet. After being on it for about six to eight weeks they were admitted to hospital for a formal double-blind challenge. The dyes used in the challenge were as shown in Table 2. Lactose was used as a placebo. Some of the doses of the dyes were small, but when the study was started we felt that these were the maximum amounts of each substance that a child would have at any one meal. There were considerable variations; for example, a glass of orange may contain between 0.5 and 1 mg of tartrazine per glass, and fish fingers may contain up to 100 mg of sunset yellow. The capsules used

Table 2 Azo-dyes and additives used for the challenge

Lactose placebo	
Tartrazine (E102)	0.1, 0.5, 1 mg
Sunset yellow (E110)	0.1 mg
Amaranth (E123)	0.1 mg
Indigo carmine (E132)	0.1 mg
Carmoisine (E122)	0.1 mg
Sodium benzoate (E211)	100 mg
Monosodium glutamate	100 mg
Sodium metabisulphite (E223)	10 mg
Aspirin	100 mg

Note: these doses are probably well below the normal intake for
   some children

for the double-blind challenge were put in individual containers and they were code-labelled by the pharmacist. We did not know the code until the challenge was completed, neither did the parents or the child know what was in the capsule or even the nursing or medical staff who were administering the capsules. The capsules were given at regular intervals and if a child showed a reaction to one of the capsules the subsequent one would be delayed until the reaction completely subsided. During the challenge observations that were made were both objective and subjective, the objective ones being temperature, peak expiratory flow rate, respiratory rate, blood pressure and pulse. The subjective ones were scratching, difficulty in breathing, vomiting, diarrhoea and rash. These observations were made by trained nursing staff who looked after the children throughout the challenge, and the observations were made at 15-minute intervals.

Criteria for a positive reaction

The primary criteria were rash and pruritis. In the forty-three children who were challenged the presenting feature was rash and pruritis. The secondary features which were looked for were a rise in temperature of over 1°C, a 20% rise in the respiratory rate, a 20% rise in the pulse rate, a 20% fall in the peak expiratory rate, and obvious behaviour change. In this study population there were four asthmatics and all of them showed a 20% drop in their peak expiratory flow rate. The other point to mention is that in 80% of the study population who showed a positive reaction there was a rise in temperature of 1 °C, which coincided with the appearance of the rash.

Results

Of the forty-three patients, one patient showed a reaction to the placebo, eleven showed a reaction to tartrazine, twenty out of thirty-six showed a reaction to sunset yellow, four out of thirty-seven showed a reaction to amaranth, and so on. Not all the patients were challenged with all the individual challenge substances because when we started the study we used the common ones first and as we went along we started adding new challenge agents. There are altogether about 3500 food additives which are available in the EEC and all over the world, and to challenge all of them would take

Table 3 Results of the challenge

	Number challenged	Number of positive reactions
Lactose	43	1
Tartrazine	43	11
Sunset yellow	36	10
Amaranth	37	4
Indigo carmine	19	3
Carmoisine	12	0
Sodium benzoate	27	4
Monosodium glutamate	36	3
Sodium metabisulphite	12	1
Aspirin	42	1
18 children did not react to any challenge		
5 children gave positive prick skin tests to inhalants		

a very long time! Further analysis of the forty-three patients indicated that twenty-four of them showed a positive reaction, some of them reacting to more than one challenge substance. One showed a placebo response and eighteen showed a negative response. The latter children went back onto a normal diet after their challenge and were followed up for about twenty-four months, and none of them subsequently relapsed or had any other symptoms. The diets of the children who reacted were modified depending on the substances to which they reacted. Twenty-one of them did not subsequently relapse but three did, and this may be because there had been a slip-up in the diet or they may have reacted to some other substance which we did not test for, or else the dose which we used for the challenge was not adequate.

Following open demonstrations of an adverse reaction to foods, a double-blind challenge of artificial colourings can therefore help to identify those ingredients not likely to cause reactions. Partial or complete relaxation of the strict diet depending on the challenge response did not result in relapse in the non-responders, thus avoiding the unnecessary imposition of a prolonged diet.

Conclusion

This trial looked at one aspect of food colouring sensitivity but it is common to find multiple symptoms occurring in affected subjects. It is fairly easy to identify dermatological manifestations which lend themselves to doing objective challenges, but when it comes to less objective central nervous system manifestations such as behaviour change, moodiness etc., such challenges could be extremely difficult to use to identify the offending agent. Another reason may be that some of the additives could be naturally occurring in foods and to produce objective results it may be necessary not only to control the absolute amounts of additive but also the form and frequency with which it is ingested.

REFERENCES

Supramaniam, G. and Warner, J. O. (1986). Artificial food additive intolerance in patients with angio-oedema and urticaria. *Lancet*, **2**, 907–909

10

How infant allergies can lead to behaviour and learning problems

D. Rapp

Some children cannot learn or behave appropriately because they have unsuspected and unrecognised allergies. The information in this chapter will share some observations that have been made by some physicians which should help you to recognise whether your child has this type of problem or not. Some allergy specialists are now able to reproduce sudden changes in activity, behaviour or the ability to learn by using deliberate food challenges or newer diagnostic methods of allergy skin testing.

Many parents are distraught by the way their children act and behave. They are disappointed because their children do not seem to be able to learn in a manner that is commensurate with their intellectual capabilities. They don't understand why their child acts like Dr Jekyll, and then suddenly, within moments, switches to Mr Hyde. It is often easy to figure out the answers (Rapp, 1979*a*, 1980, 1986). Let's discuss how this can be done.

Keep records of what a child eats *before* sudden changes in personality or ability to learn. Simply omit a suspect problem food from the child's diet for four days (Randolph, 1981; Rapp, 1979*a*, 1980), then purposely feed that food to the child, and see if the child's symptoms or personality changes recur within one hour. The answer may have been found. If the offending food is then eliminated from the child's diet, no medications are needed. The bottom line in medicine must be a method to help eliminate a child's symptoms, not to mask them with appropriate drug therapy. Many of the suggestions included in this chapter will enable parents and health educators to do exactly that.

Many children who have unusual allergic manifestations can be recognised by their appearance (Rapp, 1979*a*, 1980, 1986). For example, it is not unusual to see an allergic child who has hayfever push his nose up toward the ceiling with the heel of his hand or rub his nose vigorously because it itches (Figure 1). If a youngster does this, it usually indicates nose allergies. Affected children often have dark circles or puffy bags under their eyes. When I first began to diagnose this problem I saw a 5-year-old black boy in our hospital clinic. His eyes were almost slits. He had been told at a hospital allergy clinic that he

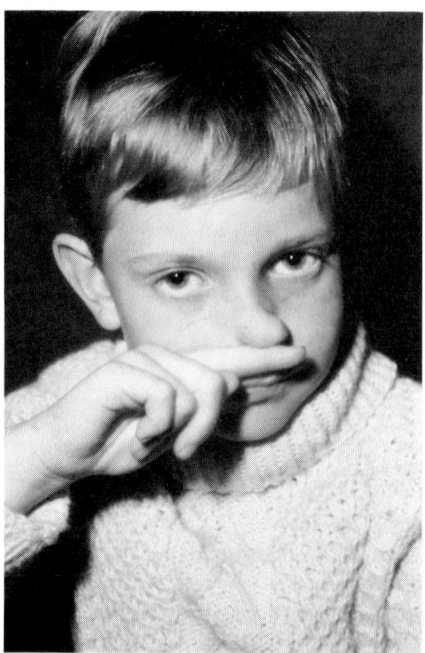

Figure 1 Characteristic facial mannerisms of allergic children. (Used with permission of Dr Verrier Jones, Landough Hospital, South Glamorgan.)

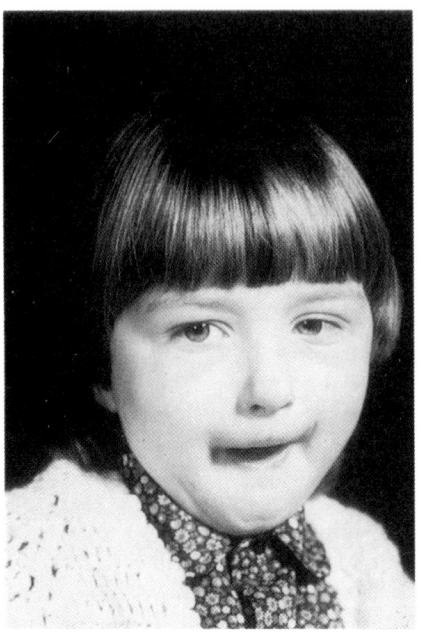

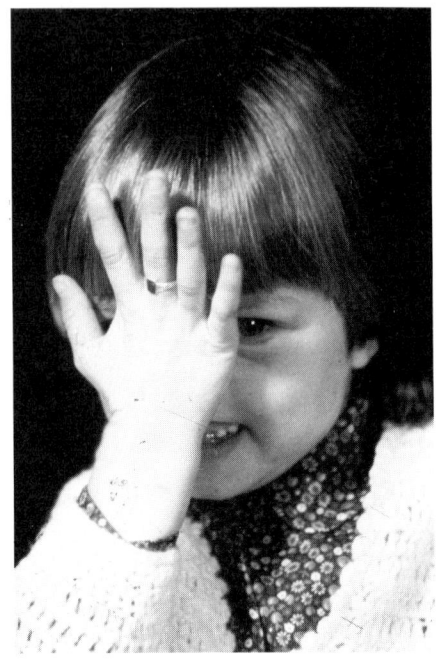

did not have any allergies. His favourite food was milk. When dairy products were discontinued, his eyes markedly improved within one week and within two weeks he had no vestige of puffiness below them. One must wonder how many other children have swollen eyes because of a favourite food. It is interesting that the typical allergy skin and blood tests (RAST) used to diagnose milk allergy were negative.

Another youngster in a hospital ear clinic was seen because he had had tubes (these look like a tiny piece of straight elbow macaroni) placed through his ear drums approximately seven times. The tubes would stay in place for several months and then fall out. They were repeatedly replaced so that the youngster did not develop a hearing impairment because of recurrent fluid formation behind his eardrums. He had extremely dark eye circles. His bedroom was made more allergy-free and his diet was altered. This chronic ear problem subsided completely. In spite of his allergic appearance and typical allergic family history, he, also, had negative allergy skin tests. He responded well to treatment that did not entail either skin testing or allergy injections. Some youngsters respond quickly and easily, provided their parents are willing to make changes in their home and life-style.

Other physical characteristics which could indicate an unsuspected allergic reaction are bright red ear lobes and wiggly legs (Rapp, 1979a, 1980, 1986). These changes are noted especially in children who have hyperactivity, behaviour or learning problems. The younger children who are hyperactive, irritable, aggressive or silly, in time often tend to become tired, fatigued or depressed adolescents.

In the 1930s, Albert Rowe described a condition called 'allergic toxemia' (Rowe, 1959), in the 1940s, Theron Randolph called it 'allergic fatigue' (Randolph, 1947) and in the 1950s Frederick Speer similarly described the 'allergic-tension-fatigue syndrome' (Speer, 1954). Many children (or adults) with this problem have classical nasal allergies, with sniffling, sneezing-in-bouts, nose rubbing, stuffiness or watery nose mucus. In addition, however, patients with the allergic-tension-fatigue syndrome tend to have some combination of the following symptoms (Rapp, 1979a, 1986):

(1) They may be tense and hyperactive, or fatigued, irritable or depressed, at times to the point of suicide.

(2) Their tongues may be unevenly coated and appear to have islands of bald patches.

(3) They find that their ability to read, write, draw, colour, or think is erratic. Sometimes they do well in school; at other times their performance is inexplicably poor.

(4) They frequently complain of headaches and muscle aches (particularly leg aches).

(5) They wet the bed after the age of 5 years, need to urinate frequently and have to rush to the bathroom.

(6) Many can't get to sleep, stay asleep or get up in the morning.

(7) They have disposition problems, i.e., they cry easily and are moody, sullen, withdrawn or aggressive.

(8) The intestinal symptoms include halitosis, belching, burping, bloating, nausea, vomiting, diarrhoea, constipation and even soiled underwear.

All children, of course, do not have all these complaints. If an individual has an allergic family, personal allergies such as asthma, hayfever, or hives, and an allergic appearance, it certainly does suggest that the types of medical complaints that were just listed could represent an unsuspected allergic reaction. Everyone must be extremely careful, however, not to think that every physical complaint is caused by allergy.

Parents often ask how they can tell the difference between a normally active youngster and a hyperactive child (Rapp, 1979a, 1986). Normal children play games. The activity of hyperactive children is purposeless, such as racing through halls and running in circles. They frequently have glassy, glazed eyes and a spaced-out look. Their ears and cheeks may become bright red and they have dark eye circles. During these hyperactive periods they are frequently either aggressive or unbelievably silly. When anyone sees sudden Dr Jekyll/Mr Hyde personality changes in a child who has been asked to do something or reprimanded, ask one important question: What did that child eat, touch or smell within the past $\frac{1}{2}$–1 hour which was different? The answer may have been found.

It is sometimes possible to trace hyperactivity in a child all the way back to the uterus (Rapp, 1986). It is not unusual for mothers to say that the baby kicked so hard that she was in tears, or her ribs were black and blue because the baby hit her so hard, from the inside, when she was pregnant. Some mothers describe the babies as 'punching their way out of the uterus'. Others say that the babies hiccuped so frequently that they had major discomfort. Excessive hiccups and vigorous moving are two ways that an unborn baby can give a mother a message. These clues should alert mothers to recognise the cause of the problem. It is frequently something the mother ate. Sometimes the offender is a chemical odour which the mother smelled. Odours cause problems within fifteen minutes or so. Foods appear to cause problems within minutes to a few hours after a pregnant mother eats a problem food.

When mothers are asked about their diet during that period, we often find that the mother loves or craves milk, yogurt, ice-cream or cheese. Many pregnant women eat more dairy products than normal during their pregnancy. Other mothers absolutely hate milk, but they drink it because they believe this ensures they'll have a healthy baby. These mothers not only make themselves ill, but they may help their unborn baby to develop a milk sensitivity. After birth, milk or dairy products can trigger hyperactivity during the infant, toddler or childhood period and possibly later on. This can occur both in breast fed infants of mothers who drink an excessive amount of cows' milk or eat too much cheese or ice-cream, or in the babies who drink a cows' milk formula, if cows' milk is a problem.

Please don't get the impression that only milk and dairy products cause infant distress. Some mothers, who have an increased awareness about this sort of cause and effect relationship, have noted other foods (i.e., bananas and chocolate) or that chemical odours can trigger unusual agitation in the womb. It is easy to confirm that the same exposure often causes similar symptoms before and after a baby is born.

After birth, youngsters destined to be hyperactive often continue to hiccup frequently and they definitely are more restless and wiggly than most babies. They may not sleep all night until they are over 3 years old. These are the infants who have to be held when you reach for a diaper or they roll off the table. They can walk at 7–10 months, rather than 12–15 months. They tend to break the crib as they rock it from one end of the room to the other, or they can bang their heads so hard that their foreheads are bloody, black or blue.

Many normal infants have colic for two or three months, but allergic colic can last for many months. They pull their legs on their belly and they scream, not only later in the day, but at times for twenty out of twenty-four hours. These infants tend to be unhappy and irritable. The distressed mothers often switch the infant's formula from milk to soya. Sometimes this helps, but some babies continue to have difficulty because soya or corn is also a problem (dextrose). These infants often have a stuffy nose, or a rash on their cheeks and outer lower arms and legs. Recurrent ear infections under the age of 1 year are not uncommon. This is particularly associated with a milk sensitivity. Allergic infants may be most reluctant to smile, for months or years. It is always gratifying and surprising to note that a simple one-week diet can change some of these unhappy babies and youngsters into bubbly, delightful darlings in a few days (Rapp 1979a, 1980, 1986).

Infants who have unrecognised allergies often perspire so much that their clothing has to be changed several times a day. They may drool so much that they need to constantly wear a body length bib or their socks are wet. Some mothers have to change the infants' sheets and put dry towels under the babys' heads during the night because they are so wet from excessive drooling or perspiration. All babies perspire and they drool when they teethe, but infants with unrecognised allergies can manifest these problems to an extreme degree.

It is not unusual for some allergic breast fed infants to have no problems until they are given cows' milk at 9 months or so. Within a month or two many of the previously outlined symptoms suddenly appear. This suggests that the youngster is sensitive to dairy products. One clue to this problem is the infant who repeatedly pushes away the bottle, but eats food vigorously. Some infants seem to realise that milk is a problem.

Toddlers present problems which are somewhat different from those in infants (Rapp, 1979a, 1986). Frequently they complain of leg aches. Mothers have to rub their legs in the middle of the night or these youngsters will suddenly lay down in a shopping mall and state they can't walk. Physicians often interpret these complaints as growing pains. Milk sensitivity, in particular, frequently causes this specific problem and the exclusion of dairy products for a week before reintroduction can clearly demonstrate if a cause and effect relationship exists.

The 'terrible two's' are notorious for temper tantrums (Rapp, 1979a, 1986). Some children have up to twenty tantrums a day and other children have one constant episode that begins in the morning and continues well into the night. Some of these episodes are abnormal brain responses to the ingestion of certain foods or to allergenic exposures to pollen, moulds, pets or chemical odours. These children tend to bite younger siblings, parents, the furniture, toys or themselves. They champ their jaws, hit, spit, kick, pinch and punch. Other toddlers refuse to get dressed or continually take off their clothing. Others cannot sleep and have repeated nightmares. Some refuse to be cuddled and have never been held in anybody's arms because they dislike being touched. These problems can be intermittent or constant. Some of these children vomit clear mucus and retch when they eat. This suggests a milk sensitivity, but other foods cause similar symptoms. Some youngsters in this age group are excessively fatigued, sleep too much, and cannot play as long as other children. Allergic toddlers also can perspire and drool more than normal. Others have one infection after another. Sometimes these complaints are secondary to an undiagnosed or untreated allergy. Many affected children also have sneezing fits, an itchy nose, and either a stuffy nose or the watery nose mucus so characteristic of hayfever. In contrast, children with infection usually have green or yellow mucus and a fever and other family members are also ill.

Children with these types of complaints can be skin tested using newer methods so that it is possible to reproduce the child's exact symptoms with one dilution of an allergy extract and to eliminate it with another dilution. However, the doctor must be familiar with the more precise newer methods of testing. It is also important that the parents do not know about the item being tested, to help eliminate bias when the results of testing are interpreted.

Let me discuss two typical youngsters. Linda had problems from early infancy, with itchy rashes and prickly heat. She drooled much more than normal as an infant. She began wheezing before 1 year of age, shortly after she ate oats for the first time.

On one occasion we wanted to confirm the type of response that this youngster could have from an injection of one drop of an allergy extract of milk. Neither Linda nor her mother knew what was being tested. The first injection of a non-allergenic salt solution caused no change in her behaviour or personality. The second injection contained a drop of milk that had been diluted 125 times. Within ten minutes she became a screaming, totally uncontrollable child. She was then given two drops of a solution of milk allergy extract that was diluted 15 000 times, and within seven minutes she was happy, normal and well-behaved. The newer types of allergy testing can produce and eliminate symptoms of this type at will, and clearly pinpoint the specific causes of some youngster's behaviour and personality problems (Rapp, 1980, 1986). Many parents and physicians are sceptical about these methods of testing, but there seems to be no doubt that these observations can be reproduced at will by those who have expertise with the newer allergy testing techniques (Rapp, 1986).

Another patient was $4\frac{1}{2}$ years old when he was initially seen. His mother was concerned because his behaviour was so uncontrollable and unpredictable that she had no idea where or if she could place him in a school in the fall. His IQ was 81. Since he had been a toddler he had been hyperactive, impulsive and aggressive and he spat, kicked, hit, punched, bit, refused to wear clothes and had inexplicable Dr Jekyll/Mr Hyde episodes. He had tantrums and at that time he had a spacey look, dark eye circles, and puffiness below his eyes. In addition, he drooled, had halitosis and his abdomen was bloated. He had ear infections repeatedly.

He was placed on a Multiple Elimination Diet (Rapp 1979a, 1980, 1986) and his response was dramatic and rapid. Within three days he acted in an almost unbelievably consistent and acceptable manner. By the end of seven days he could sit, write and even cut with scissors. His mother could not believe he was the same child. He spoke coherently and in sentences. He no longer attacked his mother. He stopped racing impulsively down the street and was pleasant and cooperative.

During the second week of the diet, the potentially allergenic foods were added back, one at a time. Within twenty minutes after he was fed wheat, the child's total personality changed. He was attacking the dog, babbling, spitting and trying to eat a plate. He was uncontrollable. His reaction to the reintroduction of milk into his diet was so violent that he put his head through a glass window. His gastro-intestinal symptoms recurred. When he was subsequently allergy skin tested for these items, his personality, writing and drawing changed dramatically. Figure 2 clearly shows how he wrote and drew prior to an allergy skin test for wheat, which is found in bread, cake, cookies, etc. After a placebo injection for an item which caused no allergy he draws, writes and acts the same. The response to the wheat skin test, however, was clearly evident, not only in his writing and drawing, but also in his marked deterioration in his behaviour within a few minutes.

Within nine days after appropriate allergy extract therapy his mother estimated that he had improved 50%. Within six weeks he was 95% improved. He could eat most foods on a four-day rotation, except for wheat. He had to avoid this food in any form for many months, but he can now eat it without reacting in any manner. His IQ, six months after this allergy treatment was begun, increased to 110. He is now 7 years old and is in an advanced reading class, takes preliminary geometry and algebra, speaks Spanish and is starting to learn Japanese. The medical complaints and behavioural problems which were so evident at $4\frac{1}{2}$ years are no longer evident, *unless* he discontinues the use of his allergy extract.

This child clearly illustrates the dramatic changes which can occur in children who have unsuspected allergies. Their response to appropriate therapy can be most gratifying for all concerned.

Other children can act similarly. Figure 3 shows a drawing by a 3-year-old prior to the time that he was tested for milk. Ten minutes after he received two drops of milk diluted 625 times he was irritable, crying and whining. His drawing at that point was merely a scribble. A few minutes after receiving one drop of milk diluted 25 times he became happy and playful again. His drawings reflected the marked change noted in his personality during testing.

Parents can determine if a food is affecting their child in an adverse manner by merely having the child draw a picture or write prior to eating. Ask the child to do it again fifteen to thirty minutes after eating. If there is a marked change, some item in the previous meal might be a factor interfering with that child's ability to learn.

Drawings and Handwriting Changes In 5½ Year Old Robert

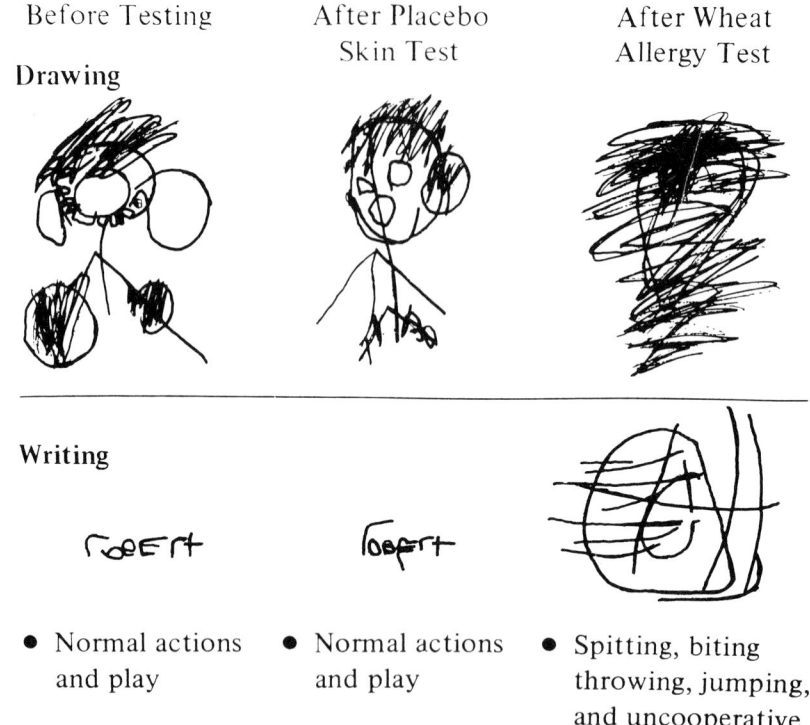

Before Testing	After Placebo Skin Test	After Wheat Allergy Test
Drawing		
Writing		
• Normal actions and play	• Normal actions and play	• Spitting, biting throwing, jumping, and uncooperative

Figure 2 Test with wheat allergy extract. (Reproduced with permission from Rapp and Bamberg, *The Impossible Child*)

In Figure 4 6-year-old Sarah's writing appears normal prior to being tested for strawberries. She was tested for these because her parents had noticed that she became hyperactive when she ate them. During the testing she began to write upside down *and* began to read from the right to the left, instead of the left to the right. After she was given the correct dilution of strawberry, she could again write and read normally. How many other children might have learning problems in school because of unsuspected food sensitivities?

Any allergic medical complaints can occur in any age group, but a few seem to be especially evident in adolescent youngsters and adults. The latter often appear to be extremely tired and irritable. They are more apt to have emotional outbursts of crying or hitting, rather than hyperactivity and biting. Older children tend to complain of recurrent headaches, muscle aches, intestinal problems, depression and the fact that their heads feel ballooned or fuzzy. They may say it feels creepy and crawly under their skin. Sometimes they are nervous and their joints ache. They often intermittently dislike any form of physical contact or touching.

Sometimes a simple one-week exclusion diet and making the bedroom of toddlers, children and adolescents more allergy-free will relieve many of the

Changes In Drawing Of A 3 Year Old Boy

| Before Test | During Test | After Milk Treatment |

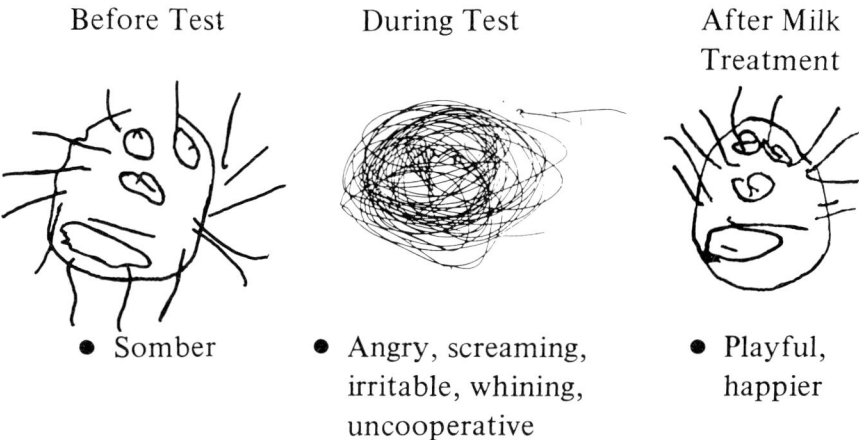

- Somber
- Angry, screaming, irritable, whining, uncooperative
- Playful, happier

Figure 3 Test with milk allergy extract. (Reproduced with permission from Rapp and Bamberg, *The Impossible Child*)

symptoms just described (Rapp 1979a, 1980, 1986). Sometimes the problem is as simple as removing a feather pillow or quilt or stopping all dairy products. The medical complaints that these children have are often mis-interpreted as psychological problems by doctors and friends, when actually there is a definite physical basis for the problem.

Basically, if you have a sore on your foot caused by a nail in your shoe the answer is to remove the nail, not to put a bandage on the sore (Rapp, 1980). In medicine there is a tendency to treat most illnesses with medicines or drugs to relieve the symptoms. Specialists in environmental medicine believe that much more time should be spent by everyone to try to determine *what is causing the illness*. Elimination of the cause is preferred to treatment of the effect. Everyone must ask themselves why a particular individual is having difficulty in the morning and not in the afternoon. Why is that person ill on a particular day, in contrast to some other day? What did that individual eat, smell or contact which might be different or unusual? Could an item or odour be contributing to that individual's not feeling well? Everyone has to increase their awareness. Instead of taking another pill, they should sit down with a pencil and paper and try to record the specific circumstances which preceded the onset of a particular medical complaint. If this is done it is often easy to figure out its exact cause.

One needs only to reason logically and know a few basic facts to determine exactly what is causing some allergies (Rapp, 1979a, 1980, 1986). In general, the causes of allergy are as follows:

(1) It is something outside the home.

(2) It is something inside a person's home (school or work area).

6 YR. OLD SARAH'S WRITING
(HYPERACTIVE AFTER EATING STRAWBERRIES)
BEFORE STRAWBERRY TEST.

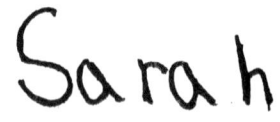

BASELINE

WRITING DURING STRAWBERRY TEST
(AT THIS TIME SHE READ BACKWARDS,
WAS UPSET, UNCOOPERATIVE, WITHDRAWN
AND IMMATURE)

AFTER 0.05cc 1–625 STRAWBERRY

WRITING AFTER STRAWBERRY
ALLERGY TREATMENT

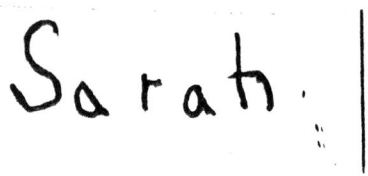

AFTER 0.05cc 1–5 STRAWBERRY.

Figure 4 Test with strawberry allergy extract. (Reproduced with permission from Rapp and Bamberg, *The Impossible Child*)

(3) It is a food.

(4) It is a chemical.

This is how to figure out which is causing the problem.

(1) *Is it something outside the home?* If an individual is worse out of doors from the time the trees begin to develop leaves until the leaves fall to the ground and the symptoms recur every year during approximately the same weeks, it is most likely that the problem is due to pollens or moulds. Such patients are generally better during the winter months because they are indoors, unless their home is damp or mouldy.

(2) *Is it something inside the person's home (school or work area)?* If someone seems to be ill all year round and the symptoms tend to improve when that individual goes camping, away on holiday or is in a hospital, this is an indication that that person could be ill because of house dust, family pets or moulds within his home. Such individuals feel fine when they leave their home for some reason for several days. After they return home, within one to twenty-four hours they are sick again. If this occurs repeatedly, it clearly indicates that there is something in the house that is bothering them. A detailed study should then be made to find out which room in a house seems to be problematic. For example, the individual might have to ask himself if he feels good when he goes to bed at night and worse every morning. This would indicate that the bedroom was the problem. If he always feels worse after bathing, then one must consider that the moulds in the bathroom or some body cosmetic might be the problem. If he is always worse after being in the kitchen, one should think about what was cooked in the kitchen and what food or cleaning odours might be in that particular room. If he is worse when the house is being cleaned, the problem might be stirred up dust. If he is worse in the basement, the cause might be dust and moulds in that area. A few minutes of analytical thinking and the answer is often almost embarrassingly obvious.

(3) *Is the problem due to a food?* (Egger *et al.*, 1985; Radcliffe *et al.*, 1981; Randolph, 1947, 1981; Rapp, 1978, 1979a, 1979b, 1980, 1985, 1986; Rippere, 1983; Rowe, 1959; Seely, 1985, Speer, 1954). If the individual has a problem related to a food, that person may have had feeding problems during the infant period. Teenagers might have to ask their parents if they cried frequently as infants and had to have frequent formula changes. Many individuals who have food sensitivities notice that they feel *worse* after they eat. They may be aware that certain foods bother them. They may notice that they fall asleep every afternoon after they have their favourite lunch. They may know that certain foods bother them, but for every food that they suspect, there may be several to many others that they do not recognise. Foods can affect many areas of the body adversely, but they tend, in particular, to cause intestinal symptoms such as bad breath (milk, wheat or eggs), belching, bloating, diarrhoea or constipation. The latter two bowel problems are frequently due to dairy products. When individuals belch, the food that they

73

taste is frequently the one to which they are sensitive. When the abdomen swells significantly after eating, this frequently indicates that a food was ingested to which that individual happened to be sensitive.

Surprisingly, in contrast, some people feel *better* after they eat a food to which they are sensitive. This means that they have an addiction to the food, somewhat analogous to a heroin addict who needs another injection. Temporarily he feels better, but when he needs it again he begins to feel unwell and knows that it is time for another injection. It is the same way with food addiction, first described by Randolph (1981). He explains this is merely one phase of food allergy. Some individuals must have their cup of tea or coffee, cake, chocolate, beer or candy at regular intervals in order to 'feel well'. Favourite foods, ironically, are frequently the ones which are causing an individual to remain unwell. If someone says that they love cake, biscuits, sandwiches, doughnuts and macaroni, be suspicious of wheat.

Another clue which delays the recognition of food sensitivity is that mixed messages may be noted in relation to a particular food. For example, many individuals absolutely hate milk, but they love cheese, yogurt and ice-cream. These individuals are frequently sensitive to all dairy products, but recognise only milk as an offender. If a person doesn't care less whether he eats a particular food or not, there is a greater chance that that individual is not sensitive to that item.

Food sensitivities usually occur within an hour after a food is ingested (Rapp, 1986). The symptoms can last from a few minutes to several days. In general, however, symptoms last only a few hours.

Some individuals will be worse every year during the time of year that they are eating an excessive amount of a particular seasonal food, such as peaches, tomatoes or corn (Rapp, 1986). One merely has to think about what was eaten in excess at that particular time to tell whether the medical complaints are due to a seasonal food or to pollens and moulds in the outside air.

(4) *Is the problem due to a chemical?* (Randolph, 1981; Rapp, 1979a, 1980, 1986) People sensitive to chemicals are easily recognised because they can smell odours before anyone else. They frequently know that certain odours make them sick. Similar to individuals with food allergies, they frequently either crave or detest certain odours. Once again, if they don't care one way or the other about the way certain things smell, they probably don't have a chemical sensitivity.

Many individuals who have chemical sensitivities tend to be carsick, develop headaches or become sleepy when they ride in cars, aeroplanes or buses. They often have been accidentally exposed to a massive chemical exposure some time in the past. For example, a gas furnace may have leaked, they may be repainting their house or may have been exposed to a petrol spillage. Regardless of the type of chemical, persons who are *overexposed* on one occasion sometimes notice that a very minute amount of innumerable odours, which previously didn't cause symptoms, now cause illness. Weakness, irritability, headache, fatigue, dizziness, loss of memory, and burning in the extremities are not uncommon. The challenge is to determine which odour causes trouble and to avoid that particular contact as much as possible. One must learn where that particular chemical might be found. Sometimes it is not obvious. For example, polyester clothing contains formaldehyde. Persons who are sensitised to this odour might have difficulty if they lived in a trailer or were exposed to panelling or certain types of insulation, as these routinely contain an excessive amount of this particular chemical. They also might find that the clothing section of department stores or fabric stores, which are polluted with the chemical odours from many polyester fabrics, repeatedly trigger sudden symptoms.

When someone ascertains that a particular item is a problem, the best answer is, of course, avoidance. This is easy if you happen to be sensitive to your feather pillow or bed quilt, as cotton bedding may resolve the problem. It is easy if you are sensitive to liver or squash. You can live without these foods. If, however, you are sensitive to dust, moulds, milk, wheat, sugar or eggs, it is very difficult to avoid these particular items. If avoidance is not possible, then it might be necessary to find a doctor who knows how to perform the newer allergy tests so that appropriate treatment can be given. Modern treatment often enables patients to tolerate exposure to pollens, moulds, dust and foods that previously caused symptoms, without the need for drug medication (O'Shea and Porter, 1981; Rapp, 1979a, 1980, 1986).

Many parents are concerned about milk and dairy products. We have been raised to believe that this is an essential food for proper growth and development. In essence, calcium or milk is necessary food for infants prior to the age of physiological weaning (age $1-1\frac{1}{2}$), during lactation and after menopause. Dr Oski, the chief professor of paediatrics at Johns Hopkins, has stated in his book that milk is not necessary after the age of $1\frac{1}{2}$ years *if the child eats a well-balanced diet*. Most mammals in the animal kingdom do not receive milk after they are weaned. In our society, however, milk and dairy products are routinely ingested throughout an individual's life. Cows' milk has been noted to cause irritability, colic, multiple feeding problems and the recurrent accumulation of ear fluid behind the eardrums during the infant period. In toddlers it is frequently a cause of retching, recurrent leg aches and bouts of hyperactivity. In older children it is a frequent cause of clucking throat sounds, throat clearing, a runny nose, asthma, bloated abdomen, diarrhoea, constipation and bed wetting beyond the age of 5 years. In adults it frequently appears to cause any of the previously mentioned symptoms as well as fatigue, irritability, joint pains and an irritable bowel. This list is far from complete and for obvious reasons arbitrary, but it does tend to indicate the type and scope of symptoms that can be noted in the different age groups from this one food item.

It does appear that a spectrum of typical allergic symptoms, as well as many other acute and chronic physical and emotional complaints, can at times be related to unsuspected allergic reactions. The brain is only one area which can malfunction because of sensitivities to foods, chemicals, dust, pollens, moulds and pets. The characteristic symptoms often can be traced from infancy through childhood and adolescence. Many typical physical and behavioural clues have been reviewed. Once the awareness of this possibility exists it is sometimes easy to pinpoint the specific cause of a medical problem. The ultimate answer in medicine must be elimination of the cause of an illness, whenever possible, rather than treatment with one drug after another.

In closing I should like to answer some questions that are frequently asked by parents of allergic children.

(1) *Is sublingual (under the tongue) allergy extract treatment as effective as monthly injections of allergy extract?*

In my experience it is equally effective for most individuals. It certainly does not help everyone, but it appears that the correct dilution of the item which causes allergies does tend to eliminate symptoms to such a degree that many patients do not require drug therapy. Occasionally some patients do not respond to sublingual treatment. Those individuals may respond well if the allergy extract is administered by injection. Initially, sublingual treatment is used three times a day, but after a few weeks or months of the treatment it is needed only once a day or less often. At that point the patient usually can eat more and more of the offending food or is able to be exposed to the normal amounts of dust, moulds or pollens without significant symptoms.

(2) *Does allergy environmental control, chemical avoidance, diet and allergy extract treatment help everyone?*

Of course not. It is not a panacea, but it can be piece of the pie. If an individual happens to be ill because of these items, comprehensive treatment is usually helpful. The sicker a child is, the more apt the parents are to comply with the suggestions made by the physician. However, most individuals become lax in relation to their doctor's recommendations as soon as their child starts to feel better. If a youngster has a strong sensitivity to a particular food, though, parents will usually limit the ingestion of that food item, especially when the youngster repeatedly has symptoms that interfere with normal function related to eating that food.

(3) *How helpful are diets?*

In general, if a patient is on a four-day rotary diet not only do minor food sensitivities disappear but new food allergies are thought to be prevented. Again, it is not the answer for everyone. Some patients can never eat certain foods that cause violent reactions. Other individuals find that they can eat some foods at an eight or twelve day interval, but not more frequently. In general, however, many patients find that if they eat them no more frequently than every four days, the foods which previously caused symptoms can be eaten without difficulty. This ability to eat problematic foods appears to be greatly enhanced by sublingual or injection food treatment in some individuals.

REFERENCES

Egger, J., Carter, C.M., Graham, P.J., Gumley, D. and Soothill, J.F. (1985). Controlled trial of oligoantigenic treatment in the hyperkinetic syndrome. *Lancet*, **1**, 540–5

O'Shea, J.A. and Porter S.F. (1981). Double-blind study of children with hyperkinetic syndrome treated with multi-allergen extract sublingually. *J. Learn. Dis.*, **14** (4), 189

Radcliffe, M.J. *et al.* (1981). Food allergy in polysymptomatic patients. *Practitioner*, **225**, 1651–4

Randolph, T.G. (1947). Allergy as a causative factor of fatigue, irritability, and behavior problems of children. *J. Pediat.*, **31**, 560

Randolph, T. (1981). *An Alternative Approach To Allergies.* Bantam Books, New York

Rapp, D.J. (1978). Does diet affect hyperactivity? *J. Learn. Dis.,* **11,** 56–61

Rapp, D.J. (1979a) *Allergies and the Hyperactive Child.* Simon and Schuster, New York

Rapp, D.J. (1979b). Food allergy treatment for hyperkinesis. *J. Learn. Dis.,* **12,** 42–50

Rapp, D.J. (1980). *Allergies and Your Family.* Sterling Publishers, New York

Rapp, D.J. (1985). Allergies: Are some children pains in the class? *J. School Admin. Assoc. New York State,* **16,** 29–32

Rapp, D.J. and Bamberg, D.L. (1986). *The Impossible Child – In School – At Home.* Practical Allergy Research Foundation, Buffalo, New York

Rippere, V. (1983). Food additives and hyperactive children: A critique of Conners. *Br. J. Clin. Psychol.,* **22,** 19–32

Rowe, A.H. (1959). Allergic toxemia and fatigue. *Ann. Allergy,* **17,** 9

Seely, S., Freed, D., Silverstone, G. and Rippere, V. (1985). *Diet-Related Diseases: The Modern Epidemic.* Avi Publishing Co., Westport, USA; Croom Helm Ltd, Beckenham, UK

Speer, F. (1954). Allergic tension-fatigue in children. *Ann. Allergy,* **12,** 168

11

The role of food intolerance in child psychiatry

I. Menzies

Introduction

Until recently the profession has been sceptical of the concept that environmental factors play a part in the development and maintenance of many different chronic conditions. Happily, this situation is now changing. Many recent studies have highlighted the importance of dietary factors, and the joint report of the Royal College of Physicians and British Nutrition Foundation on Food Intolerance and Aversion has given positive encouragement to the profession to seek funds for research in this area. Unfortunately, that report suggested that food and food additives did not contribute to the aetiology of behaviour disturbance and overactivity in childhood and stated, 'It is all too easy to collude with parents who cannot accept that psychosocial factors are to blame for their child's disruptive behaviour by accepting that the child is suffering from food intolerance.'

Clinical experience, now being increasingly supported by methodologically sound studies, lends support for quite the opposite view, namely, that there is on occasion too ready a willingness on the part of the professionals in many different disciplines to ascribe a psychosocial aetiology to a child's behaviour disturbance when the primary cause is often not poor parenting, disturbed relationships, or social deprivation but rather adverse responses to environmental factors. Most frequently, but not invariably, these are to food and to chemicals in food or drink.

The nature of the referrals

Chronic illness, handicap and behaviour disorders are now at the centre of paediatric care. Behaviourally disturbed and learning disordered children are common. They make great demands on parental understanding and courage, as well as on professional judgement and time. Many problems of classification in child psychiatry remain unresolved; although Rutter and others have demonstrated an emotional and a conduct disturbance variable, as well as a hyperkinetic grouping, there is considerable overlap between these groupings, particularly between the neurotic and conduct disordered groups. As a result, a mixed category has had to be included in the derived classification schemes. The majority of the cases referred to me present as mixed category problems. A search of the psychiatric literature for descriptions of disturbed and disturbing children revealed the work of Speer (1958) and others on the allergic-tension-fatigue syndrome. These authors stressed the aetiological importance of environmental factors – ingestants, inhalants and contactants – and stated that an environmental approach could often be of considerable help to such children.

Speer used the term 'tension' to embrace several different types of over-activity, both motor and sensory. Motor activity gives rise to restlessness, fidgetiness, clumsiness, tremor, jerkiness and even stuttering, whereas sensory overactivity is characterised by an oversensitivity to noise, light, scolding and correction and indeed to almost all external stimuli, physical and mental. He used the word 'fatigue', for, paradoxically, the tension-ridden child is also likely to be subject to 'fatigue not benefitted by rest'. When they are young such children are often irritable, sullen and easily annoyed by trivial incidents. They may lose any desire to play and may respond very negatively to parents. Later they may exhibit sleep disturbance with restlessness, frequent waking and disturbing nightmares. They have variable mood states, sometimes associated with compulsive behaviour and at other times with paranoid ideation, and they may show considerable destructiveness and excitement, surprising cruelty to playmates, and attention-demanding behaviour. Some chatter constantly, using a high pitched, strangely different voice. Parents also report bizarre, 'silly' behaviour, emotional lability, mental sluggishness, inability to concentrate or remember details and an incapacity on the part of the child troubled in this way to carry out instructions.

Clinical clues

The cases described by Speer and his colleagues are remarkably similar to many referred to me, for I have seen many parents who complain about their child being inattentive, on the go all the time 'as if driven by a motor', unable to sit through a meal, complete a task, listen to a whole story, follow directions or accept discipline. Learning problems often follow upon these children's short attention span and inability to concentrate, yet many are of average or above average ability. They may have associated speech and/or motor coordination problems as well as perceptual difficulties, so any learning problems that exist are made worse. Behavioural problems also develop; they may show constant or intermittent irritability, hostility, aggressiveness or depression. Such children may also talk a lot, cry excessively, seem unusually 'whiny' or throw tantrums easily. Sometimes excessive sweating, especially at night, and considerable thirst are also features. Parents often complain of a Jekyll and Hyde quality to their child's personality. Vague physical symptoms are also common. These include poor appetite, aching muscles and joints, paraesthesiae, facial pallor, infra- or peri-orbital oedema and a variable bluish/black/purple discolouration of the skin below the eyes (allergic shiners). Headache and vague stomach ache are also found, as is some degree of constipation, diarrhoea or halitosis. The child may also suffer from rhinitis, urticaria and mouth ulcers, and night wetting may be troublesome. Varying combinations of hyperactivity, learning and behaviour problems upset family, peer, and school relationships. This in turn has a detrimental effect on the child's self-image, and so begins a vicious spiral of trouble for child, family, school and community.

Aetiological factors

Environmental factors should be considered especially when the child and his family show many of the following features:

(1) Where the parents seem concerned, capable and interested and where the marriage relationships appear normal.

(2) Where the child had received reasonable amounts of love, attention and affection and where siblings are making satisfactory progress.

(3) Where there is a family history of allergy, migraine and/or of food or chemical intolerance and where the child's diet is markedly skewed towards refined sugar, white flour and additive-containing products.

Some of these children are diagnosed as hyperactive in that they suffer from a condition which begins early in life, is more common in boys, and is manifested by a symptom pattern of hyperactivity, impulsivity, distractibility and excitability, with also, perhaps, emotional and antisocial behaviour, specific learning problems and emotional lability complicating the picture (see Chapter 8). These problems may be on the increase. The Assistant Masters and Mistresses Association recently reported a worrying increase in incorrigible school entrants, aged 4 and 5 years. A variety of explanations is being offered for this phenomenon, particularly the influence of television. So far the possibility of adverse effects of food and/or chemicals in food has received little attention. The prognosis for untreated hyperactive children may be quite poor. Antisocial behaviour is often severe in the adolescent hyperkinetic child. A study in 1971 of a group of such children showed that more than half had been involved in fighting, stealing and destructive behaviour and two-thirds were considered incorrigible by their parents, more than one-third had threatened to kill their parents, 7% carried weapons, 15% were fire-setters, and 15% were already excessive drinkers by the age of 16. Both retrospective and prospective studies indicate that antisocial behaviour, educational retardation, depression and psychosis are prevalent in many such children as 'grown-ups'.

The role of nutrition and other environmental factors in the aetiology and treatment of behaviour problems and learning difficulty in childhood is interesting as these problems have not obviously lessened either in frequency or severity in recent years although the birth-rate has fallen. The distress and the disability caused to child, family, school and community by emotional, intellectual, and educational handicaps exceeds the distress and disability caused by physical handicap. Despite advances in child care techniques and the introduction of behaviour modification, family therapy and other approaches, our therapeutic cupboard remains somewhat empty! Psycho-dynamic understanding does not always lead to effective management, so we must be careful lest we foreclose on investigations or add an additional burden simply by applying a psychiatric label. That way, important environmental factors will remain hidden, their importance unrealised.

Our clinical experience has shown that food intolerance and chemical sensitivity frequently contribute to the problems of children suffering from a wide range of emotional, behavioural, habit and learning disorders and so since 1979 we have been looking clinically at the hypothesis that 'some of these problems may derive, at least in part, from abnormal reactions to foods and to inhalants in certain genetically predisposed, sensitive people, whose body homeostatic mechanisms have been disturbed by a variety of stresses, emotional as well as physical'.

Treatment strategies

In our child psychiatric clinic we have used simple environmental and 'allergic' management regimens to treat many of our routine cases, as the techniques are safe and non-invasive. The regimen often includes a programme of house-dust mite management, combined with carefully supervised dietary changes, including the elimination of a variety of additives as well as, on occasion, avoidance of one or more foods. More conventional methods of management are still very much in evidence, for we see no dichotomy between the psyche and the soma. Indeed, we believe that our emotions can strongly influence our body's immune and other defence mechanisms both positively and negatively.

I work closely with an extremely skilled social worker whose work with a proportion of the referred cases is both central and crucial, yet, where necessary, she will initiate or support environmental aspects of case management. Environmental screening is undertaken as a first step in most cases. These approaches often produce a substantial improvement. Moreover, relapses, when they occur, are all most always easily traced and found to be linked entirely to either non-compliance with the treatment regimen or to the inadvertent exposure of the patients to probable incitants.

Oligo-antigenic diet treatment is difficult to apply and not without its hazards. Unsupervised diets can be dangerous, more expensive and at times somewhat disruptive to family life. Skilled dietary advice should be available on an ongoing basis. However, much can be achieved simply by improving a child's nutrition and by reducing his 'chemical load'; for example, by cutting down on the amount of highly processed products he consumes, especially those which contain large quantities of refined sugar and chemical additives such as the artificial colourings, flavourings and preservatives, most of which are manufactured from either North Sea oil or coal, and by encouraging mothers to keep their houses, their laundry and themselves as free as possible from non-essential, highly scented products such as air fresheners, perfumes, polishes, detergents, fabric conditioners and the powder some sprinkle on carpets before vacuuming. There is no gainsaying the fact that often this approach has transformed family life for the better to an extent far beyond that which would have been achieved using more established therapeutic approaches.

Therapeutic problems

Treatment should be attempted only if the child seems willing and if the parents understand the rationale, are capable and motivated and have the necessary resources. Children are likely to have problems with the food and the chemicals which they most crave. For as long as they continue to eat the problem foods every day the source of the symptoms is masked and so the problem is likely to remain unresolved. If the offending substance is removed and then reintroduced between the 5th and 12th day after elimination the ensuing adverse response is most evident. Incidentally, there is growing evidence that behaviour may also be adversely influenced by pollens, house-dust mites, perfumes and gas fumes, in certain sensitive children. Any trial of an additive-free diet should last for at least three weeks, and friends, neighbours, teachers and school nurses can easily sabotage the attempt. If possible the entire family should embark on the regimen together, for the trial is unlikely to succeed if the affected child is singled out and made to feel different. Initially the child's problems may become worse rather than better because of the withdrawal effect. Artificial colourings and flavourings in items such as toothpaste, 'plaque' disclosing tablets and medicines should not be used for the period of the trial. Environmentally-induced illnesses tend to be polysymptomatic and multisystem in character and may involve chemicals in air and water as well as in food and drinks. The onset in children can usually be related to major stress factors such as the birth of a sibling, infant feeding difficulties, parental separation, or, on occasion, a viral or other infection.

Clinical examples

Hamish, aged 6, typifies one end of the spectrum of my practice, whilst Michael, aged 9, illustrates the other. Hamish was a catarrhal child with a history of croup, mouth ulcers, morning grumpiness and excessive sweating at night; he was also hypersensitive to noise and to smells. A few weeks after an attack of chickenpox and a further flu-like illness he became deeply depressed and began to talk about death and dying, much to his parents' distress. He recovered completely and quickly when free-standing butane gas heaters were removed from his environment both at home and at school but became psychotically disturbed when challenged with butane gas and its combustion products. Michael had been referred by my neuropaediatric colleague for the treatment of intractable, severe, recurrent headaches of longstanding. These cleared completely after exclusion of wheat and chemical additives from his diet. He remained free from headache except when given a pie at school. Yet his past medical history included tuberculous meningitis, complicated by porencephalic cysts, hydrocephalus, precocious puberty, hemiparesis and epilepsy!

Robert, the elder of two brothers, aged 7 and 4, had been referred because of behaviour problems. His parent's marriage had been short-lived and stormy due to his father's difficult personality. However, when seen, his mother had the support and help of a much more stable and supportive man. Robert's birth was normal, he was bottle fed, and as a young child he suffered from croup and from earache. He also complained frequently of headache and was restless, fidgety and had a short attention span and poor concentration. At times he had difficulty in expressing himself clearly, although it was obvious that he understood all that was said to him. His mother felt that he often seemed a sad boy, easily frustrated, and prone to tempers, especially when he was having difficulty saying what he wanted to say or when he was having problems with his homework. At these times he had often been aggressive and on one occasion had even taken a knife to his brother's fingers. Mother and Robert both reported substantial improvement in their headaches and in their other symptoms once their diet was free from milk and dairy products; otherwise, they stayed locked in periodic conflict and hate.

John, aged 6, is typical of the majority of the children I see. He had long presented medical problems to his increasingly distressed mother. Initially a cuddly, well behaved infant, his symptoms began at the age of 18 months, shortly after the birth of his brother. He could not be disciplined, had massive temper tantrums and was often stubborn and wilful. At times his mother could get him to respond only by suggesting that he did exactly the opposite to that which she wished. He was overactive, ill-coordinated, restless and fidgety, had no age-appropriate sense of danger, cried easily and for little reason, was hypersensitive to smells and inclined to do silly things. He was allergic to penicillin, had frequent right earache and from time to time developed headaches. He looked pale and had peri-orbital swellings. His brother and father suffered from asthma, and mother was a tense, anxious, phobic lady whose sleep was often disturbed and who frequently had feelings of unreality. Treated as a food and chemical sensitivity problem by the elimination of chemical additives and milk and dairy products from his diet, John improved dramatically, but relapsed when challenged. Robert and John are not unique, there are many like them around.

Susan, aged 6, an adopted child, had given her parents great joy for the first three years of her life. Her behaviour had been unremarkable and she had displayed no eating or sleeping problems. Following the arrival of her baby brother, also by adoption, the situation changed dramatically. She became increasingly overactive, restless and fidgety and lacked concentration. Emotionally labile, she exhibited severe temper tantrums and was very aggressive towards the baby and her parents. She also refused the family's food, skewing her diet increasingly and quickly in the direction of junk foods containing chemical additives, refined sugar and white flour. By the time of referral this situation had existed for nearly three years and the emotional atmosphere in the house was very fraught, especially at mealtimes. Despite her appearance, careful nutritional analysis showed that her diet was inadequate in a number of respects. Biochemical investigation revealed a vitamin B1 and B6 deficiency. When her nutritional problems were corrected her behavioural difficulties resolved.

Dietary factors can be important in other ways. Thomas, aged 6, an only child of a single parent, lived in an isolated farm cottage and therefore had been very eager to start school, but found himself excluded for almost two-thirds of his first year on account of soiling. He had been seen by his headmistress, the school doctor, the family practitioner, the social worker, two psychologists and a paediatrician before being referred. Enquiry revealed that he had looseness of bowel rather than soiling but only during the afternoons of school days. His mother, however, had noticed even before he started school that Thomas had looseness whenever he ate oranges, grapes, or a well-known brand of tinned beans, or drank coca-cola. Suspecting the school dinners, I suggested that Tommy should have only bread and jam with water at lunchtime, for the family ate well each evening. The problem ceased and did not return. For me it was an important case, for if there is even one child in each primary school suffering from a gut hypersensitivity problem, but diagnosed as encopretic, then that is one per school too many.

Recent Research

In research studies, Egger and his colleagues have made two most important scientific contributions to the nutritional approach. The conclusions of their first paper, entitled 'Is migraine food allergy? – a double blind controlled study of oligo-antigenic diet treatment', were as follows: '93% of 88 children with severe, frequent migraine, recovered on oligo-antigenic diets. The causative foods were identified by sequential introduction and the role of the foods provoking migraine was established by a double blind controlled trial in 40 patients. Most patients responded to several foods; many foods were involved, suggesting an allergic rather than an idiosyncratic, i.e. metabolic pathogenesis. Associated symptoms which also improved in addition to headache included abdominal pain, behaviour disorders, asthma and eczema.' The second and, to my mind, pivotal paper, 'Controlled trial of oligo-antigenic treatment in the hyperkinetic syndrome', was summarised as follows: '76 selected over-active children were treated with an oligo-antigenic diet. 62 improved and a normal range of behaviour was achieved in 21 of these.' (See Chapter 8.) These findings have raised the important question as to whether diet might be effective in a wide range of conditions even when patients come from very socially deprived backgrounds. Perhaps some of that very deprivation has had its roots in food sensitivity in other family members, for there is no doubt that these problems are familial.

The role of food chemicals

What is the relevance of behavioural toxicology to overactivity and learning disabilities, and is there any connection between the chemicals in our food and the growing number of overactive/behaviourally disordered and learning disabled children? My belief is that overactivity and perhaps even other forms of cerebral disturbance may stem from a lack of inhibitory processes in the central nervous system and that some of the oil- and coal-derived chemicals increase irritability and lessen impulse control in much the same way as do glue, other solvents and alcohol. The United Kingdom has approved a greater number of artificial colours than almost any other industrialised country. For example, the UK has approved seventeen, the EEC has approved twelve, the USA has approved seven, and Norway has banned all artificial colours.

Behavioural toxicology and other adverse effects of tartrazine (E102) in a substantial minority of people are already well recognised, as are similar responses to other artificial food colours (see Chapter 9). Amaranth (E123), a red dye, is allowed in most foods and is often used in convenience foods such as packet soups and sauces, tinned fruit, jam, ice-cream, cake mixes, biscuits and yogurt. In France and Italy it may be used only in caviare. Erythrosin (E127) exerts a significant effect on neurotransmitters in synaptosomal preparations. If this is also true *in vivo*, then noradrenalin might be reduced and disinhibition increased. Interestingly, the effect of ritalin is to increase the noradrenalin availability and so a calming effect is generated. Erythrosin is also a potent photosensitiser and one wonders whether some children may be suffering from the effects of substantial quantities of the dye becoming photosensitised as it passes repeatedly through the retinal capillaries.

Feingold suggested that natural salicylates could provoke hyperactivity and other problems. Swain *et al.* recently investigated 140 children with urticaria. Eighty-six improved substantially using elimination diets, and almost 75% reacted to double-blind challenge with salicylates (see also Chapter 9). A number of authors have pointed to the role of phenolic food compounds in environmental medicine. They believe that a high level of petrochemical hydrocarbon contaminants, more specifically phenols, creates excessive stress on the enzymes which handle the phenol ring food compounds and other phenol substrates and so an inhibition of production of these enzymes occurs, which interferes with the metabolic handling of these foods.

Modern mechanised commercial handling of vegetables, for example potatoes, can greatly increase their phenol content compared to that found in the same variety carefully looked after and gently handled. Perhaps, therefore, modern food processing methods in this way place an added strain on the subconjugation mechanisms for phenol. Sulphoconjugation by phenolsulphotransferase (PST) is an important pathway for the metabolism of a wide range of substrates; for example, monoamines and their metabolites and many phenolic drugs and presumably other phenols. These are soluble enzymes widely distributed and found in plenty in platelets and in the gut. Two forms exist: PST/M and PST/P. Two recent studies are therefore of interest. Adams *et al.* examined the stools of nine hyperactive children and twelve control children for phenol content and found that although there was no difference in the phenol levels the P-cresol content on average in the hyperactives was significantly higher than in the controls. P-cresol is the end product of tyrosine and therefore may reflect an excessive intake of milk. Attention has been drawn already to the excess milk consumption pattern in chronic delinquents. The presence of large amounts of P-cresol in the gut of a hyperactive child is cause for concern, especially if the condition is chronic. Moreover, the amounts of phenols in faeces are no indication of the amounts that may be absorbed and escape detoxification, possibly to act on the nervous system. An important next step would be to show P-cresol in the blood of hyperactives. Free P-cresol generated by gut flora is rapidly conjugated in the body, predominantly with sulphate, a metabolic step which facilitates urinary excretion. The enzyme involved, phenolsulphotransferase (PST-P) has P-cresol as a specific substrate. Gibb *et al.* have now shown that certain food and drink constituents are potent and specific inhibitors of platelet PST *in vitro*. Catechins are found in many common foods, including tea and cocoa. They inhibit PST-M to a lesser extent and exert only a negligible effect on the other monoamine degrading complex, the monoamine oxidases. Red wine strongly inhibits both forms of PST, with a greater effect on the P form, as do anthocyanins, the natural pigments responsible for the colour of many fruits and vegetables. Synthetic food colourants, especially carmoisine (E122), erythrosin (E127) and amaranth (E123), are also potent inhibitants of PST-P *in vitro*. Tartrazine, on the other hand, has virtually no effect. It is hypothesised that if any of these 'active' compounds or some of their breakdown products with similar inhibitory ability were to reach a high concentration within the gut they might prevent the subconjugation of P-cresol, thus bringing about increased circulatory concentrations of the free, potentially toxic compounds.

Future Recommendations

What, then, are the recommendations which emerge from the above confused and complex situation? Schauss points out that the study of nutrition and its effect on human behaviour is in its infancy and makes a plea that the many variables and interrelationships between diet and behaviour should not overwhelm physicians and scientists. He believes that the food industry should support all objective efforts at assessing the subtle and not so subtle effects of today's food technology on behavioural and cognitive function.

As a first step we should accord as much attention to the biological and physical as we currently now give to the psychological and social for, clearly, if the diet can affect children's cognition and behaviour, as now seems the case, the topic should have priority for scientific scrutiny. Recent moves towards snack school meals should be carefully reviewed, as should the availability of 'junk foods', dilute-to-taste drinks, and penny tray sweets in school tuck shops.

The role of the dietitian and the nutritionist in child care must be afforded a much higher priority, for within a team structure they can often make greater and more lasting improvements in the child and his family's function than can the psychiatrist, psychologist or social worker. Indeed, I suspect that nutritional problems may well underpin many of the so-called 'allergy and intolerance' problems. All child psychiatric patients under the age of 12 and certainly those who are still preschool should be screened, even if only in the most rudimentary of ways, for evidence of food intolerances, chemical sensitivities and poor nutrition. Similar opportunities should urgently be made available to children currently 'in care'.

Easily understood information about chemical additives or residues must be made freely available, to enable diets to be more easily adjusted towards healthier living. Unless absolutely indicated, artificial colourings, flavourings and preservatives should be used only if the manufacturers themselves and the Government can prove that they are not harmful to health. Moreover, behavioural toxicological approaches must feature in future determinations of these substances' safety.

Conclusions

The argument as to whether these problems are or are not immunological is a sterile one. Undoubtedly some are, although only a few are clearly IgE-mediated. In these the total IgE is high and there is evidence of atopy and of IgE specific RASTs. In other patients, immune mechanisms probably still operate, as there is evidence of eosinophilia, total immune complex excess, complement cascade abnormalities and even, occasionally, of abnormal T and B cells. Some cases are probably linked to heavy metal intoxication, whereas others may be due to vitamin and mineral deficiencies. At times essential fatty acid problems may cause trouble. I have dwelt at length on the toxic pharmacological effects of oil- and coal-derived chemicals, especially the azo-dyes, phenols and salicylates, for these make a major contribution. There may be other factors of considerable importance; for example, the role which Candida plays has been stressed by some and also the place in the atmosphere of chemicals such as the hydrocarbons, the phenols, ethanol and formaldehyde, to mention only a few, for these are likely to have impact in this area, and finally, we must assume that many tap-water supplies are bacteriologically clean but chemically polluted (see appendix 1).

Surely, there can be little doubt about the need for a truly multidisciplinary scientific approach to the elucidation of these complex multifactorial problems, for they clearly demand a multifaceted solution. Perhaps such research requires a different strategy, at least initially, for the complexity of data and the number of interacting variables suggest that there is a need for both 'computer assistance' and techniques of synthesis as well as for the more established methods of analysis. I believe such endeavours will have far-reaching implications for the assessment and treatment of disturbed delinquents and learning disordered children and their families.

REFERENCES

Adams, R. F. *et al.* (1985). High levels of faecal P-cresol in a group of hyperactive children. *Lancet,* 7 December, 1313

Alun-Jones V. *et al.* (1985). Crohn's disease; maintenance of remission by diet. *Lancet,* 27 July, 177–80

Bellanti, J. A. (ed.) (1984). Editorial in the Fifth International Food Symposium of the American College of Allergists. *Ann. Allergy,* **52** (6)

Feingold, B. F. (1976). Hyperkinesis and learning disabilities linked to the ingestion of artificial food colours and flavours. *J. Learn. Dis.,* November

Gibb, C. *et al.* (1986). Inhibition of phenolsulphotransferase P by certain food constituents. *Lancet*, 5 April, 794

Lawrence, J. and Steed, D. (1985). Primary school disruption. *J. Assist. Masters and Mistresses Assoc.*, September, 4–5

Lessof, M. H. *et al.* (1980). Food allergy and intolerance in 100 patients – local and systemic effects. *Quart. J. Med.*, New Series XLIX (195), 259–71

Lockey, S. D. (1977). Hypersensitivity to tartrazine and other dyes and additives present in foods and pharmaceutical products. *Ann. Allergy*, **38**, 206–10

McGovern, J. J. *et al.* (1983). Natural foodborne aromatics induce behavioural disturbances in children with hyperkinesis. *Int. J. Biosoc. Res.*, **4 (1),** 40–2

Mendelson, W., Johnson, N. and Stewart, M. (1971). Hyperactive children as teenagers: a follow-up study. *J. Nerv. Ment. Dis.*, **153**, 273–9

Monro, J., Brostoff, J., Carini, C. and Zilkha, K. (1980). Food allergy in migraine; study of dietary exclusion and RAST. *Lancet*, **ii**, 1–4

Rapp, D. J. (1979). *Allergies and the Hyperactive Child.* (New York: Sovereign Books)

Ratner, D. and Vigder, K. (1985). Juvenile rheumatoid arthritis and milk allergy. *J. Roy. Soc. Med.*, **78**, 410–13

Rea, W. J. and Mitchel, M. J. (1982). Chemical sensitivity and the environment. *Immunol. Allergy Practice*, **4** (5), 157–67

Royal College of Physicians and the British Nutrition Foundation (1984). Food intolerance and food aversion. *J. Roy. Coll. Physic. London*, **18** (2)

Schauss, A. G. (1985). Nutrition and behaviour. *J. Appl. Nutr.*, **35** (1)

Schauss, A. G. (1985). Research links nutrition to behaviour disorders. *School Safety*, **3**, 20–8

Selmer, J. C. and Staudenmayer, H. (1985). The practical approach to the evaluation of suspected environmental exposures; chemical intolerance. *Ann. Allergy*, **55**, 665–73

Speer, F. (1958). The allergic-tension-fatigue syndrome in children. *Int. Arch. Allergy*, **12**, 207–14

Swain, A. *et al.* (1985). Salicylates in foods. *J. Am. Diet. Assoc.*, **85** (6), 950–60

12

Diagnostic methods for food intolerance

A. J. Franklin

In many areas of medicine today clinical diagnoses can be confirmed or refuted by the use of appropriate laboratory tests. The problem with food allergy is that there is no definitive diagnostic test.

A clinical diagnosis is based on the assessment of the patient from a good clinical history which relates exposure to symptoms. Sometimes this is established by the exclusion of alternative confirmable diagnoses. As we have noted in earlier chapters, it may also be established by clinical improvement when the relevant substance is avoided and relapse when challenged, preferably several times and preferably using a double-blind technique. Alternatively, histological changes in the bowel mucosa may be observed following challenge but this necessitates a biopsy technique. Unfortunately, these methods are not always possible and never easy to do in ordinary clinical practice, especially in small children. The earlier discovery of IgE antibody as the 'reaginic' substance responsible for allergic reactions led to the development of the radioimmunoassay and later the enzyme-linked assay of these specific IgE antibodies to inhalant and food allergens. The early promise of a reliable *in vitro* test for food allergy has been disappointed by the poor correlation in practice of positive IgE with clinical reactions. Clearly, not all food intolerance is immunological, even though the symptoms and signs may be similar. For example, lactose intolerance due to deficiency of lactase and cows' milk protein intolerance (allergy) both present with diarrhoea and failure to thrive in infants fed on cows' milk. Both improve when milk is withdrawn and both relapse on challenge, but the distinction can be made by lactose challenge and only a small proportion of cows' milk allergic infants produce measurable specific cows' milk IgE. Different fractions of cows' milk protein may act as the allergen in different individual patients and several fractions may operate together in others. Radioactive labelling has been used experimentally to follow the course of some of these protein fractions.

Whatever the mechanism of intolerance, the patient only wants to know what to avoid to return to normal health. If we concentrate only on immunological reactions (true allergy) we shall only succeed in helping about one-quarter to one-third of our patients. As we saw in Chapter 1, sometimes several of the mechanisms operate simultaneously and the level of symptoms may rise and fall with the emotional state of the patient, as it does in asthma. Food intolerance is a complex disease involving immunological, inflammatory, toxic and psychological mechanisms.

Is it therefore reasonable to seek for a single simple test for food intolerance? I submit that it is not and that the first requirement is to become familiar with the different kinds of reactions to foods that are commonly seen. As Pearson and Warner have pointed out, patients can be sincere yet mistaken about foods making them ill and this can have serious implications for a child whose parents deprive him of foods in the mistaken belief that he is reacting adversely to them.

Review of methods of testing for allergies

A good dietary history

A history of food intake, quantity and frequency and a note of any reactions which the patient may have been conscious of following ingestion are absolutely fundamental to a diagnosis of food intolerance. In children this should include early feeding history, whether breast fed or which formula was used, how the baby fed, whether he settled after feeds or spent much time with colic and crying, the amount of thirst which the young child demonstrated, and reactions to the first introduction of weaning foods. A note should be made of any development of allergic symptoms in any system of the body soon after first exposure to a new food. Note should also be taken of taste reactions – avoidance or craving for particular foods – and relation of symptoms to infection. Screening for infection or thrush should be undertaken at this stage.

Skin prick tests

This simple 'office' procedure (not universally well tolerated by small children) can be quite misleading for, as with the RAST, some tests may be positive but not correlate with the foods taken, and some negative despite clear responses to challenge. Tests may remain positive long after the food has ceased to cause problems. As Frankland has demonstrated, fresh antigenic material may react quite differently from freeze-dried preparations, which are often used for testing. The advantage of skin prick testing is that it is a quick procedure and a large number of antigens may be tested on the skin at the same time. Dr Lingam described a child with bad breath who had been extensively investigated with negative findings. Skin prick testing suggested a positive reaction to cheese which, when avoided, cleared up her symptoms.

A small drop of the food extract is placed on the skin and a small amount of the fluid is introduced into the epidermis by gently lifting the skin with the tip of a needle or pressing a small plastic pointed stick through the drop into the skin using a special device, the Morrow-Brown test needle. This is often much more acceptable to children than using a steel needle or metal pricker.

The resulting positive weal and flare response should be compared with control solutions of glycerol saline and histamine.

Patch testing

Patch testing on the skin has been used for many years by dermatologists looking for contact sensitivity. An American physician has used an adjuvant with food solutions to enhance the penetration of antigen, but each food seems to need a different concentration and the test is still being evaluated. It cannot yet be recommended as a reliable test.

Intradermal tests

These can produce very variable responses according to the dilution used. In some cases the responses can be very alarming and resemble anaphylactic reactions but the strength of the reaction may not correlate with the severity of the symptoms on oral challenge for reasons explained in earlier chapters of this book. This method is the basis of the neutralisation provocation method. Serial dilutions of the test solution can be used to find the precise point at which symptoms can be blocked or neutralised, and that concentration will then be taken and used in a therapeutic solution given by mouth. This method is both expensive and time-consuming and requires a large stock of solutions to be available for testing a range of antigens.

Sublingual testing

This method has also been used but found to be not totally reliable. Food extracts are placed under the tongue for one minute and then washed out of the mouth and observations are made on the taste reaction, for example, sweet, sour, bitter, salt or dry, creamy or burning, and on any more distant symptoms which may occur in other parts of the body.

The pulse test

This test, which was described by Coca and Cott in 1942, depends on a rising pulse rate following the ingestion of an allergic food. At least one general practice in Southampton has found it of value in adults but in children it is more difficult because of other factors, for example, mobility and emotions which affect the pulse rate. The observation should be made with the patient at rest at half-hourly intervals for up to two hours after ingestion. A pulse increase of 20% or more is thought to be significant.

Hair analysis

One UK laboratory claims to demonstrate food allergy by swinging a pendulum containing the hair sample over a food extract. There seems to be no scientific basis for this method and it cannot be recommended. Duplicate samples from the same patient under different names have given quite different results and the law of probability may operate here, even assuming that there is total honesty in reporting results. Methods and machines relating to the production of microvoltage electrical currents on the skin where they are placed near offending foods have been developed but no reliable scientific work has been published to substantiate the claims made about them. Likewise, methods of kinesthesiology, where uncontrollable transient muscle weakness indicates food intolerance as the food is brought into contact, also lack scientific evaluation, but a number of individual practitioners have found such methods quite useful for screening purposes.

In vitro blood tests

Total IgE and RAST.
Total IgE indicates the production of non-specific IgE antibody and by itself is of little value. RAST, which is more specific, is limited to a number of common foods but again it correlates only with immediate sensitivity reactions which appear within one hour of exposure and with circulating IgE, in contrast to tissue-bound IgE. Most patients are clinically aware of such reactions. Also, in several studies reported in the 2nd Fisons Food Allergy Workshop 1983 it was demonstrated that RAST positive results were dependent on the food material that was causing the symptoms being on the test disc but digestion sometimes changed the antigenic material. In a series of patients with clear clinical signs of food intolerance only about 15% had symptoms which correlated with positive RAST, whereas more patients had positive RAST with negative symptoms and others had symptoms with negative RAST. Food colourings, a frequent cause of symptoms, especially in children, are not normally amenable to testing by RAST. This is an expensive test and has really little value in food allergy.

Histamine release from basophils.
This is a research measure which has been used to indicate biological activity of a patient's cells though it gives no indication of increased localised reactions. Only about 55–60% of children with eczema gave positive results with food antigens. In cases of asthma, pretreatment with histamine can enhance some of the results. The test is a measure of systemic sensitisation and may have some value in food allergic disease, particularly when the target organ is not the gastro-intestinal tract. Heparinised whole blood is incubated with food extracts diluted in phosphate buffered saline and, after centrifugation, histamine is measured in the supernatent plasma, compared with the total available histamine.

The Bryan leucocytotoxic test.
This test, described by Black in 1956 in America, measures the degree of destruction of a patient's neutrophils when exposed to food extracts on a microscope slide. The mechanism is unknown but, like measuring IgG4 antibody, it depends really on whether the food has been eaten recently. The test requires a great deal of skill and experience on the part of the laboratory in order to get reliable and reproducible results. A major criticism has

regarded inconsistencies shown between different samples on the same day and between different observers, but further work is planned to try to improve on the reliability of this test which has potential for being a useful routine one. Up to fifty foods can be screened at one time on a single microtitre well slide. A fasting blood sample is taken and centrifuged and the buffy coat is then suspended in the patient's own serum before being added to the slide and incubated. The slide has been previously coated with food extract. The number of lysed cells is assessed biologically under direct vision and the result depends on careful technique. New electronic scanning methods may possibly make this test more useful. Experience of using the test with present techniques would suggest that the more extreme reactions frequently do indicate foods to which the patient is showing some intolerance, and foods which do not react at all can be safely used in an elimination diet. The problem really lies in the rather large group of intermediate foods which have to be excluded and challenged in the more tedious, previously described way, by dieting.

Other tests appear from time to time. Pointers to allergy may be obtained by noting blood eosinophilia or IgA deficiency but these are not specific in any way to food allergy. Intestinal biopsies following challenge are limited, as described in Chapter 2, by the possibility that the lesions are patchy and it may be a matter of pure chance whether the right piece of tissue is taken. Endoscopic vision of the stomach wall following ingestion may also be used but would appear to have limited application.

As none of these laboratory tests can be relied upon to give a clear and unequivocal answer to the question 'What is the patient allergic to?', we still seek such a test to avoid the long and tedious elimination and challenge diets, whose limitations have been already discussed and which are the only other methods available. The limitations of elimination diets have been pointed out in Chapter 1.

Elimination and challenge diet

With an elimination diet the foods to be tested are completely withheld from the patient for five to twenty-eight days, depending on the investigator. Sometimes a 'few foods' diet may be used, in which case a deprivation period of fourteen days is usually chosen, but it may take up to twenty-eight days for all the symptoms from the previous diet to settle. In cases where there is addiction, withdrawal symptoms causing an exacerbation of symptoms may appear after two to three days following elimination of the food. These must be allowed to settle before reintroduction or challenge is commenced. Failure to wait or too rapid a reintroduction may confuse the issue by masking, that is obliteration of the withdrawal symptoms by the use of excess antigen. After elimination has been instituted and withdrawal symptoms (if any) have settled, foods are challenged by reintroducing normal portions of simple foods on an empty stomach, daily for three or more days. Only one or two foods per week can be tested in this way. When looking for immediate reactions foods can be tested daily but delayed reactions may overlap if this is done in every case. On the other hand, too long a delay in challenging may allow time for tolerance to occur and subsequent challenges will then be less obvious.

Perhaps more work is needed to evaluate the place of some of the more uncertain tests described, and perhaps a combination of methods may be more valuable. The constantly changing clinical pattern of food intolerance makes the whole area into a quicksand into which the unwary can easily fall and get lost. In the last analysis, if a food taken by a patient causes unwanted symptoms, whatever the mechanism, that food is probably best avoided unless the patient is happy to live with the symptoms and in so doing avoids permanent harm. Many forms of food intolerance are transient and repeated rechallenge is necessary if very restrictive diets are to be avoided. Dietetic control is vital and desensitisation experience is still limited but may provide another option (see Chapter 17).

Summary

1. There is no totally satisfactory test for food allergy.
2. It is essential to take a good history, including a dietary history, and relate this to the patient's symptoms.
3. Establishment of an allergic diathesis may be worth while – measure total IgE, differential white blood count, IgA level, carry out skin prick test for one or more positive reactions.
4. Consult a dietitian to institute selective elimination and challenge diet or a few foods diet followed by more extensive challenge.
5. If facilities are available, consider other diagnostic measures such as RAST, leucocytotoxic test, pulse test or double-blind challenge using specially prepared capsules or food mixtures.
6. Consider the possibility of mineral deficiencies in a person on an inadequate diet. Minerals of clinical importance include iron, calcium, zinc, magnesium and manganese, and, rarely, copper, chromium and selenium as well. At the same time one may wish to look at toxic levels of minerals such as lead, aluminium and cadmium. Methods are available in some places, based on blood, sweat and hair analyses.

Note: Most NHS hospitals can do routine blood counts, total IgE and RAST tests. Many hospitals and some general practitioners can perform skin prick tests and they are available at nearly all allergy clinics. Mineral analyses and vitamin levels may be done by some NHS laboratories but the leucocytotoxic test is available only from York Medical and Nutritional Laboratories, 126 Acomb Road, York, YO2 4EY, or Larkhall Laboratories, 225 Putney Bridge Road, London SW15 2PY. Mineral and vitamin assays are also available from Biolab, The Stone House, 9 Weymouth Street, London W1N 3FF.

REFERENCES

Aas, K. (1978). The diagnosis of hypersensitivity to ingested foods. Reliability of skin prick testing and the radioallergosorbent test with different materials. *Clinical Allergy*, **8**, 39–50

Bahna, S. L. and Gandhi, M. D. (1987). Reliability of skin testing and RAST in food allergy diagnosis. In R. K. Chandra (ed.). *Food Allergy.*

Benson, T. E. and Akins, J. A. (1976). Cytotoxic testing for food allergy: evaluation of reproducibility and correlation. *J. All. and Clin. Immunol.,* **58**, 471–6

Black, A. P. (1956). A new diagnostic method in allergic disease. *Pediatrics,* **17**, 716–23

Bryan, W. T. K. and Bryan M. P. (1969). Cytotoxic reactions in the diagnosis of food allergy. *Laryngoscope,* **79**, 1453–72

Chua, Y. Y., Bremner, K., Llobet, J. L., Kokubu, H. L., and Collins-Williams, C. (1976b). Diagnosis of food allergy by the radioallergosorbent test. *J. All. and Clin. Immunol.,* **58**, 477–82

Coca, A. F. (1943). *Familial Non reaginic Food Allergy.* (Springfield, Ill.: Charles C. Thomas)

Coca, A. F. (1956). *The Pulse Test.* (New York: Lyle Stuart)

Fallström, S. P., Ahlstedt, S., and Hanson, L. A. (1978). Specific antibodies in infants with gastrointestinal intolerance to cows' milk protein. *International Archives of All. and Applied Immun.,* **56**, 97–105

Firer, M. A., Hosking, C. S., Hill, D. J. (1981). Milk-specific antibody measurement by ELISA: development of an assay. *J. Immunol. Methods,* **46**, 31–40

Gandhi, M. D., Bahna, S. L. (1985). Skin testing versus oral challenge in food sensitivity. *J. Allergy and Clin. Immunol.,* **75**, 205

Kletter, B., Gery, I., Freier, S., Noah, Z., and Davies, A. M. (1971c). Immunoglobulin E antibodies K milk proteins. *Clinical Allergy,* **1**, 249–55

Lehman, C. W. (1980). The leukocyte food allergy test: a study of its reliability and reproducibility. Effect of diet and sublingual food drops on this test. *Annals of Allergy,* **45**, 150–8

May, C. D. (1976). High spontaneous histamine release in vitro from leukocytes of persons hypersensitive to food. *J. All. and Clin. Immunol.,* **58**, 432–7

Miller, J. B., (1972). *Food Allergy. Provocative Testing and Injection Therapy.* (Springfield: Charles C. Thomas)

Osrath, P., Markus, M. (1968). Diagnostic value of thrombopenia and iosinophilia after food ingestion in children with milk and egg allergy. *Acta Paediatr. Acad. Sci. Hung.,* **9**, 279–84

Pearson, D. J., Rix, K. J. B. (1983). Food allergy: How much in the mind? A clinical and psychiatric study of suspected food hypersensitivity. *Lancet,* **1**, 1259

Radcliffe, M. J. (1982). Clinical methods for diagnosis. *Clin. Immunol. Allergy,* **2**, 205–20

Rea, W. J., Podell, R. N., Williams, M. *et al.* (1984). Elimination of oral food challenge reaction by injection of food extracts. *Arch. Otolaryngol.,* **110**, 248–52 (1975)

Shiner, M., Brook, C. G. D., Ballard, J. *et al.* Intestinal biopsy in the diagnosis of cow's milk protein intolerance without acute symptoms. *Lancet,* **2**, 1060–3

Soifer, M. M. and Hirsch, S. R. (1975). The direct lasophil digranulation test and the intracutaneous test: a comparison using food extracts. *J. All. and Clin. Immunol.,* **56**, 127–32

Wilson, N., Silverman, M. (1985). Diagnosis of food sensitivity in childhood asthma. *J. Roy. Soc. Med.,* **78** (Suppl. 5) 11–16

Wraith, D. G., Merrett, J., Roth, A. *et al.* (1979). Recognition of food-allergic patients and their allergens by the RAST technique and clinical investigation. *Clin. Allergy,* **9**, 25–36

13

Diets of children attending an allergy clinic

*M. Savage**

Over many years of nursing I developed an interest in allergies and their likely causes. Whilst studying for a nutrition diploma four years ago I chose to look at possible nutritional causes of allergies and their effects on children. I looked at thirty-six children, aged from 8 months to 15 years, with a mean age of $3\frac{1}{2}$ years, who attended Dr Lingam's clinic at King George Hospital, Ilford. As a midwife I had never considered intra-uterine movement in connection with the mother's diet. Whilst doing the project this subject raised the question of when allergies began.

The initial nutritional assessment usually took approximately two hours but some took longer. This flexibility I felt was essential, for many mothers were tired and anxious, from dealing all day and night with a child who possibly did not sleep for many hours and then only for short periods, and worried about the adequacy of their children's food intake. The mothers agreed to keep a food diary for two months and then to meet and discuss the findings. The following table shows an example of a diary on a typical day.

Table 1

Emotions	Food and drink	Body/skin behaviour
8 am Irritable on waking	Porridge with milk and sugar	Eyes red and itchy
11 am Noisy/angry	Drink	Complains of lights hurting eyes
1 pm Very difficult	Chicken Potatoes and Carrots	
3 pm Naughty and screaming	Fruit drink	Complains of pains in stomach

Many of the mothers had noted which foods appeared to make their children worse and had automatically stopped these foods. I introduced these

* Mrs Savage is the co-author of a book of diets and recipes for food allergic patients, called *The Alternative Allergy Cook Book.*

mothers to a five-day rotation diet which allowed the children to have variety without creating too much of a problem for the mothers themselves.

Examples

One of the mothers spoke of the stress of a crying child which created pressure in the marriage too. This child had cried for approximately forty minutes of every hour from birth to the age of 10 months. Feeds were changed with constant regularity to no avail. Mother had not slept for ten days or nights as she had to keep the child occupied to allow her husband to sleep so that he could go to work. The Health Visitor suggested that they stop dairy produce and try the child on a soya product. The mother did this and yet again she did not sleep that night, simply due to the fact that she continually went to check on the child, who was sleeping soundly for a substantial period for the first time since birth! Now, at the age of 3 years, this child is splendidly happy provided the mother ensures that she does not get much dairy produce. She can tolerate some ice-cream, but only once a week. The mother found that her child needed to have at least four days between treats, but if she had had some sweets and more fruits than normal her tolerance to dairy food was reduced, as she then reacted quickly to even a little, as before, with irritability, crying and screaming which resulted in a shattered mother and a very distressed child.

One bottle fed child had frequency of micturition, which had been present since infancy until this child was 7 years old, causing great distress to her. Within weeks of changing her diet the problem ceased to exist.

Another child had alternating diarrhoea and constipation. The diarrhoea was due to constipation with overflow. It was very disturbing for this young boy, aged 7, and even now it may recur. The mother noted that rich foods such as sauces and dairy produce appeared to make the situation much worse.

Another case that really stood out for me was the mother with three children in her family suffering from eczema, asthma and hyperactivity. These children were affected badly by eggs and dairy produce and their mother had suffered from skin reactions during pregnancy. She learned that eggs were not acceptable to her first two children, following skin and respiratory reactions when eggs were introduced into their diets. She decided that no dairy produce and no eggs were to be given to her third child. One day she left the child with a babyminder, giving strict instructions as to the feeds. On return she took the child home and when taking the clothes off noticed skin eruptions, which got worse over the next forty-eight hours. Blisters formed on the child's legs, the skin of the body was very red and there was some tissue swelling with oedema. It took approximately one week for the skin to return to normal. On questioning the childminder, the mother discovered the child had been given small quantities of egg and cows' milk, with the most severe reactions.

Table 2 shows the food cravings of some allergic children. All had severe thirsts, which became noticeably less when the diets were changed. Thirst created a lot of problems for many mothers as they often had to carry drinks around on a constant basis. Both thirst and craving were markedly reduced within days of altering the diet.

Table 2   Food cravings in thirty-six allergic children

Eggs	2
Salty foods	21
Sweet foods	30
Fluids	36

Table 3   Drinks favoured by allergic children irrespective of foods eaten

Orange squash
All fizzy drinks
Lemon squash
Ribena
Other blackcurrant drinks

The thirst I thought of as the body attempting to dilute an element it found undesirable (see Chapter 8 on hyperactivity). Abnormal thirst may be a pointer to food intolerance.

Social problems of special diets

Many mothers found the special diets created a great social problem. Many had lack of support regarding diet within the family unit and often within the marriage. Relatives thought the mothers were mean not allowing their children to have citrus drinks (squashes), chocolate, milk etc., and this often caused the child to have tantrums and a family argument ensued. Many mothers found that having got their families organised to at least make an attempt to support them and the child on new diets, they then had to overcome outside influences.

(1) *Schools*   There was no choice of foods to suit the child. Taking a packed lunch often meant he had to sit in the playground to eat his lunch. That is not very nice for the child in the middle of winter, but packed lunches are now much more commonly eaten.

(2) *Parties*   Many mothers reported delivering a lovely, well behaved child to a party and some three or four hours later collecting a wild, raving, naughty child who would not go to bed and was impossible to pacify. Such a change is mainly due to the fact that party foods are often full of colourings, sugar and other additives. Many mothers decided to decline the invitations, but this only makes these children feel more aware that they are not like their friends who can eat anything. It is all very difficult for them at first, for they feel removed from their friends by their allergy.

(3) *Holidays*   These have to be self-catering, which means that the mother gets no break from cooking etc. Often Mediterranean holidays are the best, as there are lots of fresh vegetables, fruits and fish. The sun, too, appears to be of value to some of the skin problems.

(4) *Guilt*   It is amazing how many mothers felt guilty on the issue of allergies and their children. They often wondered if they had done something to

cause the problem. They needed to be reassured on this and on the child's improvement.

This project made me realise the need for education of the public and those in the primary health care field.

Allergies, intolerances and sensitivities to food are here to stay and we need to know how to deal with them. Early detection means early assistance and reduction of stress and distress suffered by so many. It was marvellous to see the children improve when the diet was altered, so simple but effective. It was also interesting to see the change in the family as the child improved. From the mother being under stress within the family regarding her attitude to the child, now the family were supporting her in the dietary changes.

Following up the children one year later, it was interesting to chat with the mothers and to hear that the children had continued to stay well. Many of them had been found to develop a tolerance to many of the foods to which they had been very intolerant the previous year, provided that they were taken in small quantities and on a rotation basis.

14

Food, diets and food allergies

R. Mattis SRD

Look at your watch, what time is it? Have you just had a meal, or are you thinking about your next meal? So often our lives revolve around meal-times and special events involving food; for example, a child's birthday party with plenty of food, or an engagement with a special dinner, and again, plenty of food. Food is a social habit!

One of the roles of a dietitian dealing with food allergy is to bring science and technology down to a practical level which patients and their family can understand. We enjoy our food, so why shouldn't our patients who have food-related illnesses?

Table 1 Common presenting symptoms

Diarrhoea	Constant colds
Blocked nose	Polyuria
Asthma	Hyperactivity
Eczema	Migraine
Rhinitis	Failure to thrive

Often a family will appear in the surgery with a collection of symptoms. They have no idea which food, if any, causes the symptoms or how it relates to their reactions.

At this point it is extremely important to establish a good relationship with your patient, especially if the patient is a child. Talk to him, not over his head. Discover his favourite foods; ice-cream, chocolate and sweets will often feature as a top priority. Time spent in the beginning leads to good relationships, which lead to better dietary control in the long term.

Once a good rapport has been established, the dietitian will begin to look at the clinical evidence for the particular diet requested by the doctor. Does any one food stand out immediately as a problem factor? Does the child need a special diet? However, before any specific diet can be given to the patient, it is important that a full dietary assessment be calculated. The reasoning behind this is that in many cases the 'normal diet' of the patient will be nutritionally inadequate.

Many patients, especially children, fill up on pies, pizzas, fish fingers,

Table 2 Common allergic foods

Colourings	Milk
Eggs	Wheat
Orange	Preservatives
Sugar	Chocolate
Fish	Yeast
Nuts	Cheese

beefburgers, cakes and biscuits, and on further questioning will not be able to remember the last time they ate fresh fruit or had fresh vegetables. One particular child I came across had a menu which was as follows:

Breakfast:	Toast and jam
Lunch:	Peanut butter sandwich
	Crisps and a chocolate biscuit
	Orange squash
Mid-afternoon:	1 packet of Wotsits
	Orange squash
Supper:	Beefburger
	Tomato sauce
	Chips
Bedtime:	1 glass of milk

On gentle questioning of the mother as to why the child wasn't given fresh vegetables, the answer came back: 'If I don't give him what he wants he throws himself on the floor, bangs his head, and refuses to eat anything. He is uncontrollable!' These are the most common symptoms of hyperactivity, so before a specific diet was undertaken we decided to try to rebalance the child's diet. This decision was taken by the team involved, as all decisions should be, with the dietitian playing a key role.

It is important that the child does not feel he is being treated differently from everyone else, which usually means, to a degree, some change to the diet of the whole family. There is nothing more prone to cause friction than a child being served one meal, while the rest of the family have something else. The less tension created within the family unit the better the compliance with dietary guidelines.

In this 'age of convenience' many parents do not know what a good diet is, so it may be necessary to take them back to basics.

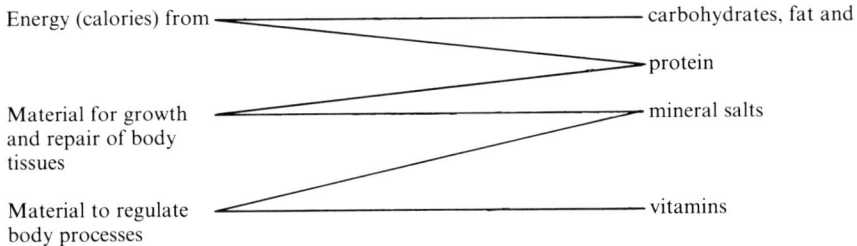

Figure 1 The balanced diet

During the Second World War diets were very much more restricted, yet children were much healthier. Parents can buy the correct food without necessarily putting a greater strain on the family shopping budget. I tend always to advise parents and patients to shop at the large supermarkets rather than the small rather over-priced health food shops.

The normal healthy diet

We encourage patients to have:

Fresh meat and fish (including oily fish)
Pulses and nuts   as a protein source
Wholewheat bread, pasta and cereals   as a source of carbohydrate
                                                                       and roughage
Fresh fruit and vegetables   as a source of minerals and
                                                                       vitamins

Excessive drinking of certain fluids may be a problem in some children, so when teaching the diet we cut out any craved drink – orange squash tends to be the main offender – replacing it with milk, fresh fruit juice and additive-free lemonade. Children should have nuts and dried fruits for snacks; sugar and junk foods should be avoided.

Often, when a child presents with failure to thrive and the paediatrician can find no clinical reason for the underlying condition, food allergy may be suspected. Check the amount of fluid consumption, for many children fill up on fluid as they don't have the patience to sit and eat.

Another area of concern can be the school meals system. Many schools now work on a help-yourself snack system, and children, being children, tend to choose chips and cakes. This can be used to our advantage in some cases; half term is an excellent time to start a healthy eating plan. Seven days at home, with records kept, then seven days at school with similar records. Our department has discovered that the 'fresh food diet' has helped to change many a child's behaviour so that instead of being an uncontrollable menace he is an attentive, interested child.

In many ways, children and/or adults with poor nutritional intakes are the simplest to help. Those patients presenting with symptoms, yet following well-balanced diets, require specific exclusion diets to be calculated.

Food allergy diets

As yet, skin and blood tests are not 100% reliable in diagnosing food allergies. They may be used as a clinical indicator as to which foods should be excluded first, but a great deal rests upon the patient's clinical and dietary history. Four different types of diet may be used as defined from the history (Figure 2).

(1) *The simple single exclusion diet* may be used when one food can be seen as the obvious culprit, e.g., strawberries, causing angioedema.

(2) *The empirical diet* (see Francis) entails the exclusion of certain foods commonly associated with a particular disease, e.g., cows' milk protein

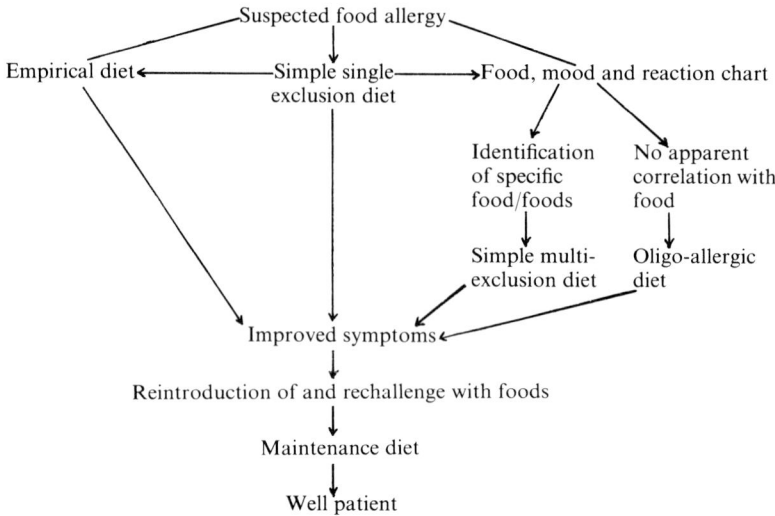

Figure 2 Scheme for diagnosis and treatment of suspected food allergy

in postgastroenteritis enteropathy (Walker-Smith, 1979), milk and egg in childhood eczema (Atherton, 1982).

The food, mood and reaction chart was formulated to alleviate some of the stress brought about by the oligo-allergenic diet. Patients have to chart the following for a period:

(a) food consumed and at what time;

(b) the mood they are in;

(c) any reaction they have and at what time.

From this chart the dietitian may be able to identify a specific food or foods which may be causing the reactions, e.g.:

Time	Food	Mood	Reaction
8 am	Blackcurrant juice	Fair	
9.15 am			Stomach pains

As people tend to eat similar things over a period of 14 days, reactions would be repeated.

(3) *A simple multi-exclusion diet* can be worked out from the reaction chart.

Table 3 Examples of offending foods

Weetabix	Eggs	White flour
Apple juice	Cheese	Cola drink
Sugar	Potatoes	Strawberry jam

Up to a total of four foods have been excluded at any one time. The process, with the offending foods excluded, is then repeated for a further fourteen days, by which time many symptoms will have improved, so that there is no need for an oligo-allergenic diet.

(4) *The oligo-allergenic diet* (Francis) should only be used if everything else has proved unsuccessful. It permits the use of only one meat, one cereal, one fruit, one vegetable, a milk substitute, Kosher margarine, salt, sugar and tea. Mineral and vitamin supplements are necessary when using this diet. It must be used only for a period of between 5 and 21 days.

The role of the dietitian

It is extremely important when teaching the specific diet that the dietitian takes sufficient time. These diets are not simple and they require more than a five-minute consultation and the giving of a diet sheet. Each diet sheet must exclude all the suspected food allergens, along with a list of manufactured foods free from these allergens. The new Government legislation on food labelling has made for easier identification of ingredients, but which busy mum really has time to read every single label?

The dietitian must be willing to be used as a resource tool, meeting the family where they are, not where we feel they should be. Helping them to plan a week's menu in advance enables the family to have suitable foods in the home. Encourage them to try new recipes and be more creative in their cookery. If the diet becomes a chore for the family, compliance is so much more difficult to establish. Some patients may even prefer the symptoms to the diet; follow-up with patience and understanding is essential.

To establish a firm diagnosis, reintroduction of the suspected allergen is essential. As the timing is critical, the opinions of all relevant workers involved in the case should be sought, and the exact timing taken as a team decision. Foods should be reintroduced in a preplanned cycle, one at a time, with a rest period of at least four days between new foods. Initially, the amount of food reintroduced should be approximately one teaspoonful. This should be given under professional supervision because of the possible risk of ana-phylaxis – working up to pre-illness intake. Apart from preventing the risk of anaphylaxis, this method may help to decide whether the food is a specific allergen or whether the symptoms are due to intolerance caused by the ingestion of excessive amounts of particular foods. If the latter proves to be the case, some workers have shown the four-day rotation diet to be useful. (This diet allows specific proven allergens to be taken in limited quantities once in four days, with little or no ill effect.) If symptoms recur on rechal-lenging, the food should be withdrawn immediately.

Nutritional adequacy of these diets is extremely important. As seen in the earlier part of this chapter, poor nutrition can cause a variety of symptoms. Therefore, as a safeguard, at least once per year a complete weighed dietary assessment should be carried out. In many ways this is how I came to be involved with allergies. Many requests for an antigen avoidance diet were received in my clinic and as a dietitian, I was quite concerned about the nutritional adequacy of this diet. Some children over the age of 2 on milk- and egg-free diets tended to dislike the various milk substitutes – were they getting enough calcium? What about their trace elements? Were they getting

enough calories? In consultation with the paediatricians and various colleagues it was decided to carry out a computer analysis of twenty-five children.
A summary of the results is as follows.

Twenty-five children were asked to complete in-depth history forms. Six
failed to do so; a further four came from socio-economic Group 5 and their
records were not accurate enough to be analysed (although from overall
review their diets looked well-balanced).

The fifteen remaining full and correct charts were analysed, with their
original presenting symptoms recorded in Table 4.

Table 4 Main presenting
symptoms of the fifteen children (seven boys and eight
girls) analysed (age range 4
months to 14 years, mean 22
months)

Eczema	7
'Short-fuse' syndrome	5
Abdominal pain	2
Diarrhoea and vomiting	2
Failure to thrive	2
Asthma	2
Papular urticaria	1
Urinary frequency	1

Some children had two presenting symptoms.

At the outset of the study each child had been on a diet for more than
three months; good compliance had been maintained, with follow-up visits
to the dietitian. The majority of diets fell into the category of egg-free and
milk-free, but other antigens (wheat, citrus, tomato, colouring and preservatives) were also excluded in some diets.

The nutrients evaluated are shown in Table 5 and the results of the analysis
are given in Table 6.

From the results shown, all children were receiving adequate amounts of
protein and calories. On individual evaluation it was noted that those children
deficient in calcium, vitamin C and iron came from socio-economic Groups
4 and 5; with encouragement they added more variety to the diets, thus
reaching the recommended daily intake. However, two children needed specific calcium supplementation.

As vitamin D was low from dietary sources in all children, it was decided

Table 5 Evaluation of food components

Protein	
Fat	
Carbohydrate	
Minerals:	Calcium, iron, sodium, potassium
Trace elements:	Zinc, magnesium, copper
Vitamins:	A, D, E, C, thiamine
	Riboflavine, nicotinic acid, folate,
	biotin, pantothenic acid, B_6, B_{12}

Table 6 Results of dietary analysis (McCance and Widdowson, 1980)

Protein	g/kg/day	Normal
Fat	g/kg/day	Normal
Carbohydrate	g/kg/day	Normal
Calories	kilocalories/kg/day	Normal
Minerals	mg/kg/day	Calcium low in 3
		Iron low in 2
Vitamins	mg i.u.	Vitamin C low in 3
		Vitamin D low in all

All compared with daily allowances for age, as recommended by:
National Academy of Sciences (U.S.A.)
FAO/WHO
DHSS RDAS

that all those put on antigen-avoidance diets should receive Vitamin D supplements.

In conclusion, it has been shown that antigen-avoidance diets can be nutritionally adequate and adapted to fit in with the normal family diet, although it does take time and careful planning to ensure the correct balance. The team approach of the doctor, dietitian, health visitor and in some cases the educational psychologist helps many families to come to terms with their allergy but it all takes time. Please, fellow health professionals, give these families the time they need!

REFERENCES

Atherton, D. J. (1982). Atopic eczema. *Clin. Immunol. Allergy*, 1982 **2,** 77–100

Francis, D. (1980). *The Proceedings of the First Food Allergy Workshop*, pp 86 and 88–9

Walker-Smith, J. A. (1979). Dietary protein intolerance. In Walker-Smith, J. A. (ed.) *Diseases of the Small Intestine in Children*, 2nd edn., Pitman Medical, Tunbridge Wells

15

Dietary management of food allergic children

A. MacDonald

Dietary therapy is difficult in every way and we should raise a number of questions before it is embarked upon. Will the diet cause more problems than the symptoms? Does a small patch of eczema on the arms or legs or an infrequent migraine attack really justify diet therapy? Are the parents capable of understanding the dietary advice or willing to persevere with it? Is the diet expensive? Special diets tend to be expensive and this can put an additional financial strain on the family budget. What age is the child? It is much easier to put a child aged 1 year on a special diet than it is to put a child of 15 years. Are there siblings? The more children there are in a family the less likely you are to keep one to a particular diet unless the whole family shares in it. Which special diets can we use? There are four main types available: simple exclusion diets, elimination diets, elemental diets and rotation diets. We find in practice that rotation diets are not particularly helpful in identifying specific food allergies. The two main ones the dietitians use are simple exclusion and elimination diets. The former eliminates a limited number of foods likely to cause the problem and the diet can be tailored to suit each case in order to confirm the clinical suspicion, especially when the reactions are obvious. For example, if a child vomits every time he drinks milk, a milk-free diet can be tried, or if he gets diarrhoea every time he eats wheat, a wheat-free diet should be tried. In this chapter I shall concentrate on only one simple exclusion diet – the milk-free diet.

The reason I have chosen this diet is that milk allergy is fairly commonly diagnosed. Although some health visitors and doctors may try to manage it themselves, professional dietetic advice is needed. Four important factors should be remembered. First, apart from the obvious, milk, cheese and yoghurt, milk is also found in many manufactured foods. Everything that contains casein, whey or lactose among other milk-containing components, should be excluded from the diet. This may include particular sweets, tinned meats, sausages, beefburgers, cakes, tinned spaghetti and soup, and patients need to be given appropriate advice on which milk-containing foods to exclude.

The second factor relates particularly to babies with suspected milk intolerance. It is not enough to switch the formula milk to milk substitute because many commercial weaning foods contain milk either in the form of casein or whey and these must also be excluded from the diet, so the mother needs advice on which weaning foods to use, or which components to look for on the labels. The most important factor is the choice of milk substitute. Milk remains an important source of nutrition for babies and small children and they need an appropriate milk substitute. Unfortunately there are many inappropriate milk substitutes available. Goats' milk and sheeps' milk are amongst these because they are particularly high in protein, high in sodium, and low in carbohydrate, so they should not be given to babies without modification. For example, to make goats' milk suitable for a child under the age of 6 months it needs to be diluted to $\frac{3}{4}$ strength and to have 5 g carbohydrate per 100 ml, vitamins A, D, C, folic acid and B_{12} added to it. Sheeps' milk is particularly high in calories, containing 100 calories per 100 ml, and should not be given to any child under the age of 1 year. If these milks come from unpasteurised sources they need boiling to prevent infection. In practice, we use neither goats' milk nor sheeps' milk. There is quite a strong cross-reaction between cows' milk and these other two milks; it is quoted that about 50% of the children who react to cows' milk would react to goats' milk as well. Health food store and supermarket soya milks are usually nutritionally inadequate since many consist only of soya beans, water and sugar or soya bean and water alone, and should not be given to babies or small children without modification.

Simple soya milk substitutes

Amongst the milk substitutes that can be given to babies and small children are Prosobee, Isomil, Formula S and Wysoy, which are based on soya protein isolate. Prosobee is the most expensive and Formula S and Wysoy can be bought directly over the counter as well as being available on prescription. If a doctor puts a baby onto soya milk for suspected milk intolerance it is important that these products are prescribed by him and that mothers do not have to buy them from the chemist, because they cost more than formula milk and would significantly increase family expenditure. Our practice is to use soya milk for babies over the age of 1 year. We do not use it for babies under 1 year because of the problems of secondary soya intolerance, which are less likely to occur in older children. For babies under 1 year of age we use either Nutramigen or Pregestimil, which are hydrolysed casein milks that have been charcoal treated to reduce their allergenicity. There is thought to be virtually no cross-reactivity between cows' milk and these two milks. Both are fine when a baby is taking from a feeding bottle as this tends to minimise the smell, but if a child has to take them from an open feeding cup it can be more difficult to persuade him to drink.

The fourth important factor about a milk-free diet is milk challenge. When we have a baby or a small child on a milk-free diet and want to challenge it with milk we never simply switch from the soya or Nutramigen/Pregestimil onto formula milk or cows' milk; we do it gradually. For example, in the first feed we would add 5 ml of normal formula to 250 ml of the soya milk or Pregestimil or Nutramigen and then would gradually increase the quantity added until we had the baby onto total formula milk or cows' milk again.

Elimination diets

An elimination diet basically involves the removal of all common food allergens from the diet for a period of two to three weeks. If there is an improvement in symptoms during this time foods are slowly and singly reintroduced back into the diet so that the offending ones can be isolated. If there is no improvement in the symptoms the diet is stopped. Patients are not kept on the diet for more than two to three weeks, as a longer period would result in poor compliance or problems with lack of calories or other nutrients. If there is no improvement in symptoms it is likely that food is not implicated in causing them, that the child has cheated, or that the basic diet still contains a food which the patient is reacting to. When, in practice, would we use an elimination diet? If the symptoms are very severe or certainly very inconvenient to the child or adult patient, and if there is something in the history to suggest that food would be implicated.

The question of which foods should be included in the basic diet is controversial, but generally most elimination diets are very much alike. We tend to include lamb, rice, carrots, pears, peaches, apricots, 7-Up, Formula S as a milk substitute, and sugar, but this is just the basic elimination diet. We do vary the diet slightly according to the conditions. For example, I have found that patients with migraine have very few problems with potatoes and other vegetables so for such patients I extend the diet and include these. For a patient with hyperactivity we might exclude some of the sugar products and include a wider range of potato and vegetables. I think the most important thing is that you start with a base of a limited number of foods. Although there may be an occasional patient who reacts to lamb or pears or whatever, we find these to be fairly low allergenic foods, and you need a basic diet to start with.

The next important point is reintroduction. Which foods first, how much of the food, and for how long? There is no agreement as to whether you should introduce food in groups or singly. We usually introduce foods singly, as we have found that this works best. For example, potatoes and tomatoes are in the same food group and we seldom find a patient who reacts to both of them. We tend to reintroduce low allergenic foods first so that the diet can be expanded without interruption, but if we have a child or patient who has a particular liking for milk or wheat, even though these are quite allergenic, we introduce them to the diet early so that the child will be more compliant. How much of the food do we introduce? Well, as a first challenge we always introduce a small amount of food on the first day and normal portions of the food thereafter. The reason for introducing a small amount of food initially is to avoid the possibility of anaphylactic reactions. For children, it has been suggested that two people should always be present on the first day to deal with such a situation but obviously this is not always possible. For how long should you introduce each food – one day, three days, or one week?

Again, our cautious policy is to introduce one food each week, as this minimises problems with delayed reactions. Interestingly, in the same patient you could get a reaction with one particular food quite severely on the first day and with another food it might take five days for a reaction to occur (see Chapter 1). We therefore tend to be fairly careful with food introduction.

Food introduction needs to be carefully supervised. It takes about a year to reintroduce all foods to the diet. I usually contact parents of children on an elimination diet weekly, certainly not longer than fortnightly, because if parents are left to their own devices for very long and they are given four to five foods to reintroduce to the diet they tend to hurry the process and will introduce them all in one go, which leads to total confusion if reactions occur. A lot of supervision is therefore needed when foods are being reintroduced.

There are various types of elimination diet in use. One example is the staged diagnostic elimination diet as reported by Hathaway and Warner. Stages 1 and 2 are types of simple exclusion diet. Stage 3 is similar to the elimination diet I have already described and Stage 4 is an elemental-type diet using a product such as Vivonex to replace all other foods. At the Hospital for Sick Children, Great Ormond Street, they use two types of oligo-allergenic diet*. Each such diet consists of one different meat, e.g., lamb or chicken, one different carbohydrate source, e.g., potatoes or rice, one different fruit, e.g., banana or apple, a vegetable, e.g., a brassica, and water with calcium and vitamins added. If the patients do not respond to the first diet they should go on to the second diet. However, with the majority of patients seen in our hospital out-patient clinics we find that after two weeks on the basic elimination diet they have had enough and are quite willing to accept that they have not got food intolerance. The patients we would contemplate putting on a second kind of elimination diet would be ones who are severely ill.

We also have an elimination diet especially for babies (not lamb, rice, carrots, etc., but Nutramigen and a milk-free baby rice). Again, an occasional baby will react to baby rice but this is unusual. Food reintroduction depends on the baby's symptoms. For example, if one of these is failure to thrive we do not reintroduce foods until some significant catch up growth has occurred. We usually find if we start reintroducing foods to the babies who have responded to Nutramigen and baby rice and have started to put on some weight, and they react to them, it reverses the weight gain and can actually put us back two steps. For this reason we do not reintroduce foods until we are getting a reasonable weight gain. This diet has its nutritional limitations but we see the patients fairly frequently to monitor growth and nutritional intake.

Problems with elimination diets

Delayed reactions

I have referred to some reactions taking up to a week. We have some patients who do not react for two weeks and with them it is more difficult to identify what is going on.

* See Further Reading list, Appendix 4.

Spontaneous remissions

We see this a lot in our migraine patients. If on the elimination diet the migraine attacks go away and six weeks later they return we may think it is the last food introduced into the diet which caused them to do so. If we take the food out and the migraine attacks do not get any better we put the patient back on to the basic elimination diet. If the headaches still continue, we may conclude that the patient had gone into spontaneous remission at the start of the elimination diet and that the headaches had nothing to do with the original diet. Spontaneous remission of migraine has been recorded.

Infections

These have already been discussed in an earlier chapter. Our children with food allergy and intolerance do tend to get a lot of infections, gastro-enteritis, otitis media, etc., and one of the problems with an elimination diet is that every time the child gets a slight infection the mother seems to think it is a reaction to the food, and we certainly have had problems with this.

Teething

Parents with a miserable, crying, non-sleeping child can easily blame food reactions, then a week later find that a new tooth has erupted. This seems to happen quite frequently.

Non-compliance

This speaks for itself.

Triggered reactions

These are something that is very difficult to prove but I am pretty sure they happen (see Chapter 1). For example, we see with migrainous children that they can eat two foods separately and not react but if they eat the same two foods in combination it will produce a reaction. Or they may be able to eat a food without reaction one day, but when they do a specific activity, such as running or playing rugby at school, then eat the same food, they have a migraine attack. These combinations are very difficult to pin-point. We usually find them more by good luck than good management but we have been able to confirm them with a few children.

The time factor

Elimination diets are very time-consuming, not only from the mother's point of view but from the dietetic point of view as well. A working mum can find it desperately hard to look after an elimination diet properly. It may mean that a nursery nurse or a childminder has to prepare the food and she may not appreciate how important it is to be careful in keeping strictly to the diet. For the dietitian it can take a minimum of ten hours to deal with an elimination diet, even without regular dietary assessment.

Cost

Elimination diets are very expensive. For a teenager aged 15 years, for example, an elimination diet would cost a minimum of £15 a week. A family on supplementary benefit would get something like £5.50 from the DHSS for a teenager and only £1.65 special dietary allowance. This is not enough to cover the cost of the elimination diet. It is possible, however, for some patients to get an allowance for a whole cost diet.

Medicines

Many medicines are coloured and it is important that patients on an elimination diet or a colour-free diet are given colour-free preparations.

Treatment changes

It is no good starting a patient on an elimination diet at the same time that other treatment is changed. For example, if a patient with eczema is referred to me at the same time that he has a new cream prescribed and there is a response, I do not know whether it is the effect of the elimination diet or the effect of the treatment change.

Calorie intake and hunger

Although children can eat any quantity of food on the elimination diet, in practice many of the older children complain that they are hungry. The migrainous children can become so hungry that they get more migraine attacks during the three weeks of the elimination diet than they have reported previously, due to the stress of hunger.

Nutritional inadequacy

The nutritional intake of dieting children needs to be checked frequently and appropriate vitamin and mineral supplements should be given.

Manufactured foods

This problem applies to both elimination and simple exclusion diets. For practicing dietitians the problem may be that there is an ingredient within an ingredient on the label. Manufacturers are under no obligation to notify these. For example, sausages frequently contain rusk. It may be that milk is contained in the rusk, but this cannot be identified by simply looking at the lists of ingredients in the sausages.

There is also a problem with the sources of ingredients. Manufacturers do not need to identify on the label whether starch is wheat or corn-based. Lecithin may be soya- or egg-based, vegetable protein may also be wheat or soya-based or it could be from any vegetable base, and animal fats may be based on butter or lard.

Munchausen syndrome by proxy

Dr Littlewood has mentioned the Munchausen syndrome by proxy in Chapter 4. This pretend allergy syndrome may be on the increase and is not helped at the moment by all the books one can buy on 'Do-It-Yourself Allergy' and media articles. It is very easy to find out what sort of symptoms you are supposed to present with and the appropriate response, and patients with non-genuine food reactions do not give food allergy a particularly good name.

Blind challenges

Finally, there is the problem of blind challenges. Frequently food allergy experts say we need to do these to prove food intolerance, but they are very difficult to do in clinical practice, as has been mentioned previously. In our clinic we do them only when we doubt the diagnosis of food intolerance, for we have not time to do them on every patient. Clearly, if a baby or young child is given a test food openly but supervised by hospital personnel and has an immediate severe reaction we do not doubt the diagnosis. Among the difficulties of performing blind challenges is how to give the food allergen. There are three basic ways: by naso-gastric tubes, disguised in normal food, or disguised in capsules. As far as the latter is concerned, there is a limit to how much of the food allergen can be put into a capsule so we tend to disguise it in normal foods.

When performing blind challenges, we like to give five normal portions of the food for about five days, but this is not always practical because of the length of time it would keep the child in hospital. Sometimes we give the child five portions of the food over the course of something like twenty-four or forty-eight hours in hospital, to see what is actually happening. Frequently, however, the children do not react in the hospital, and the parents say as they react as soon as they get home, these challenges often do not help us to decide whether a child has food intolerance or not.

In conclusion I would like to restate two important points. Children should be put on special diets for food intolerance only if the symptoms warrant it, and dietary management should always be conducted in liaison with doctors and dietitians.

16

The role of drugs in the treatment of food allergy

A. M. Edwards

Before considering the use of drugs for the treatment of allergic diseases it is important, first, to confirm the diagnosis, second, to identify the allergens that are involved in the condition one is dealing with, and third, to make a concerted effort to remove those allergens as far as practicable. This applies particularly to food allergy, for where the complaint takes the form of hay fever or, in certain cases, asthma it might not be possible to remove the allergen, but with food allergies all three steps should be carried out before one considers drugs.

Food allergy can be classified as primary or secondary: it is primary when the symptoms occur in the gastro-intestinal tract, secondary when other target organs, such as the skin or the bronchi, are involved. Most allergic reactions involve an inflammatory process at either a mucosal surface or the skin; this is not caused by bacteria or viruses but is stimulated in response to an antigen. A generalised systemic reaction can occur when an antigen is either absorbed, through the gastro-intestinal tract, for example, or injected by means of a wasp's or bee's sting.

Mechanisms amenable to intervention

A primary reaction takes place when an antigen comes into contact with mast cells in the gut; this increases the permeability of the mucous membrane and allows more antigen to pass through, thus accentuating the allergic reaction in other organs. The antibody on the surface of local mast cells releases mediators, calling in inflammatory cells, and the whole process develops into a vicious circle, which we can call the inflammation of allergy. After activation of a mast cell, the release of the preformed mediators – histamine, and others – which give the initial symptoms, is followed by the generation of secondary mediators of the allergic inflammation – prostaglandins, leucotrienes and the chemotactic factors that call in other inflammatory cells. The change in local vascular permeability, which gives rise to swelling and outpouring of fluid from the local blood system, stimulation of mucus production, increased smooth muscle contraction (which causes broncho-constriction in asthma), stimulation of pain fibres, and recruitment of inflammatory cells, leads to both immediate and late phase inflammation and also the enhancement of macromolecules across mucosal surfaces, the latter probably being the most important mechanism in food allergy.

With regard to the potential treatment of allergy by drugs, it might be possible to neutralise the antigen, for example by killing off the house dust mite or making the offending substance non-antigenic. That would be a good start and there is evidence that it is practicable. Since allergic people have IgE antibody in excess, could its production be blocked? Unfortunately, that is not yet possible, but where the absorption of food antigens through the gastro-intestinal mucous membrane can be prevented the amount of IgE produced in response to them does diminish and the sensitivity of those people to food allergy decreases. Could the release of the mediators that are involved be blocked? It is possible to interfere with the mediator production, to antagonise the mediators, and to counteract the effect of the mediators. Really, the history of drugs linked with allergy starts here and goes backwards, in that all people with allergy still have various symptoms; they have a cough and they have wheeze, if they have asthma, which can be counteracted by giving them bronchodilators or a cough medicine. The main mediator in hay fever is histamine, and this can be counteracted by an antihistamine. It is only with corticosteroids and sodium cromoglycate that one can go a further step back and either block the release of mediators or, in the case of corticosteroids, affect mediator production.

Table 1

SOME ANTIHISTAMINES USED IN THE TREATMENT OF ALLERGIC CONDITIONS
(In order of decreasing sedation effect)

Name	Trade name	Duration of action (hours)	Preparations available	Single adult dose
Promethazine	Phenergan	4–6	Inj, syrup, tabs, suppos.	25–50mg
Diphenhydramine	Benadryl	4–6	Inj, elix, caps.	50mg
Chlorpheniramine	Piriton	4–6	Inj, syrup, tabs, sustained action tabs.	4mg
Clemastine	Tavegil	6–12	Elix, tabs.	1mg
Azatadine maleate	Optimine	6–12	Syr. tabs.	1–2mg
Terfenadine	Triludan	6–12	Tabs, susp.	60mg
Astemizole	Hismanal	12–24	Tabs, susp.	10mg

OTHER DRUGS USED IN THE TREATMENT OF ALLERGIC CONDITIONS

For inhibition of prostaglandin synthesis – effect depends on the prostaglandin sub-class which predominates

Salicylate*	Aspirin	4–6	Tabs, sol. tabs.	65mg
	(larger doses may produce urticaria and bronchospasm)			
Ibuprofen*	Brufen	4–6	Tabs, syrup	400mg
Indomethacin*	Indocid	4–6	Caps, susp, suppos.	25–50mg
Mefenamic acid*	Ponstan	4–6	Caps, sol, tabs.	500mg

* May induce bronchospasm

Some allergic reactions are so dangerous that people can die from them. Whenever one is engaged in inducing allergic reactions or involved in hypo-sensitisation procedures one should always have at hand adrenaline and corticosteroids to counter the severe anaphylactic reactions which sometimes occur.

Table 1 gives some examples of antihistamines and antiprostaglandins that can be used to antagonise the mediators. It is possible, for instance, that prostaglandins are involved in enhancing the permeability of the gut to food antigens, and it has been shown in Professor Lessof's unit at Guy's Hospital that antiprostaglandins such as aspirin can interfere with this mechanism and have a therapeutic effect.

Mediators that are produced as a result of mast cell activation can be counteracted both by corticosteroids and sodium cromoglycate. There is evidence that the beta agonist group of drugs and the theophyllines also interfere with mediator production, but probably not to any great extent, so that in therapeutic terms their main effects are symptomatic on the condition rather than on mediator production. For example, in allergic conjunctivitis, one can use vasoconstrictors, corticosteroids, or sodium cromoglycate. In asthma it is more important to decide the aims of treatment. Are you aiming to just relieve the bronchospasm, to damp down the whole of the inflammatory action with corticosteroids, or to allow the person concerned to live a more normal life? Perhaps one of the things that one should do is monitor breathing patterns, by means of a simple peak flow meter. When it comes to the management of asthma with drugs, I think that one should aim to maintain people, as much of the time as possible, near to or about their normal peak expiratory flow rate. If one only takes the odd reading here or there in the surgery, the pattern is missed, and it is the way the pattern changes that allows one to control the condition by drug usage, hence the value of a peak flow meter used daily at home. Asthma these days is really a multidrug-treatment disease and it is a matter of getting the right balance of all the drugs that are available, recognising in each case how the various preparations act, singly or in combination, to produce maximum benefit.

Returning to the drug management of food allergy, I would again stress that drugs should be considered only after the main food allergens have been identified and some attempt has been made to remove them by dietary reduction. Look first at the food and where the main reaction is taking place. There is certainly a reaction in the gastro-intestinal mucosa in some cases, which can lead to symptoms of diarrhoea, sickness or abdominal pain, but it may be that the main symptoms are in the secondary target organs, which can be any organs in the body, although we tend to concentrate on the skin, the nose, the eyes and the gut. There is good evidence that the gut is also a secondary target organ and that people with allergic proctitis, and in some cases colitis, may be suffering from food allergy. The food antigen is absorbed in the jejunum, circulates round the bloodstream and causes a secondary action in the colon or the rectum. It is not the food getting down to the rectum that causes the main inflammation, it is absorption higher up.

What are the intermediate pathways? Is it a neurological reflex that is set off in one tissue and causes the symptoms elsewhere? Is it mediators that are released at the primary site that cause the symptoms? Is it an antigen that is absorbed in the jejunum or ileum which circulates around the bloodstream and sets up allergic reactions in the secondary target organs? I do not think we know all the answers to those questions, although evidence is mounting that the main problem is in the small intestine in that there is a primary allergic reaction in the gastro-intestinal mucosa which allows an increase in the absorption of food antigens. In sensitive individuals the secondary symptoms are determined by the amount of antigen that is absorbed, and the more sensitive people are the more antigen they absorb. The first principle of food allergy must therefore be to remove the antigen from the diet and only when that is not practical, or it is not known what a person is reacting to, can one look at other ways of dealing with it.

Gut absorption and Sodium Cromoglycate

Some recent work by Dr André in Lyon shows that if one measures the permeability of the gut by two sugars – and these are just markers on gut permeability – in normal subjects and in food allergy subjects who are fasting, the figures are roughly the same; but when the latter subjects are challenged with the foods to which they are sensitive the mannitol clearance falls, the lactulose clearance goes up three to four times and the ratio changes. We have shown that by pretreating these people with oral sodium cromoglycate one can bring it back to normal again. However, the principle is here, that in many cases it is only when subjects are challenged with the food to which they are sensitive that their gut permeability changes. We have been using sodium cromoglycate in its oral form for some ten years now to investigate the whole business and to see whether in fact it is a useful treatment for food allergy.

In another experiment a group of six asthmatic people, all of whom, when challenged with the food to which they are sensitive, get a greater than 20% fall in their peak expiratory flow rate, were examined by blind challenge procedures. Three were sensitive to egg, one to wheat, and two to milk. Then, in a double-blind experiment they were pretreated with either two placebos or a placebo and inhaled cromoglycate or oral cromoglycate. The results showed that we could block the asthmatic reaction which was induced by putting the antigen into the gut, by first putting oral cromoglycate into the gut, but we could not block it when we put the cromoglycate into the secondary target organ, the lung. This again emphasises that the primary reaction in food allergy is taking place at the gastro-intestinal mucosal level and is probably then enhancing the absorption of the antigen; if one can block that absorption it is helpful in the management.

The final example of where cromoglycate helped was in a group of children with eczema, all of whom were carefully selected because their condition was exacerbated when they had milk and egg. The study was done by Professor L. Businco in Rome, who had found that about one-third of all the children in her eczema clinic were allergic to just these two foods; a third had multiple food allergies and another third did not seem to have any food allergy at all. They were placed on a diet from which milk and eggs were excluded, and further improvement was obtained by adding cromoglycate to their management. They were still possibly having something in their diet which was causing them some problems, although they had really minimal symptoms, assessed on a range of symptoms from 0–12. There was some increase in symptoms when they were challenged with food whilst they were being treated with placebo, but when they were treated with cromoglycate the increase was not so great. That is why I think there is some value in using oral cromoglycate in the management of food allergic disease, but only when at least the main antigens have been removed from the diet (see also Chapter 6).

In conclusion, I return to my first point: in the management of food allergy with drugs, first confirm the patient has an allergy, secondly identify the allergens, thirdly remove them from the diet, and then and only then, if you are still having problems in the management of the patient, add in a drug such as oral cromoglycate to help to control the symptoms.

17

Immunotherapy for allergic disorders: a controversial subject

L. M. McEwen

The best kind of medicine is always conservative and if patients can manage to remain well by the simple avoidance of one or two foods then they are wisely best left alone. A little simple advice may be all that is needed. Other patients with transient or trivial symptoms may be treated easily by safe drugs or topical creams in small amounts. However, there are other patients whose lives are made either dangerous, from the risk of accidental anaphylactic reactions, or miserable by having to carefully, laboriously, or expensively, control their diet, or if they become sensitised to a large number of common foods, they may suffer from actual malnutrition, so that alternative methods of treatment are required.

Methods of immunotherapy for food allergy

I want briefly to discuss the following five alternative methods:

(1) Conventional immunotherapy by incremental allergen injections.

(2) Graded normal exposure to allergen (oral desensitisation).

(3) Neutralising therapy.

(4) Pulse steroid therapy.

(5) Enzyme potentiated desensitisation.

Conventional desensitising injections

Blackley first applied raw pollen to the abraded skin in 1865 and although he showed no improvement in his subsequent hay fever he did show a large immediate response. Noon in 1911 published an account of an injection method, which with modification has continued to the present day. Frankland in 1952 published the first double-blind trial of the method in the treatment of hay fever, and despite attempts to characterise and purify antigen extracts

125

for vaccination over the past thirty years his results still stand and have not really been improved upon. Since then, allergists have been using mixed vaccines containing pollens, foods, animal dander and mould extracts for the prophylactic treatment of allergic disease in a relatively unproved and uncontrolled way. In fact, most of the attempts to produce double-blind controlled trials with these vaccines have failed to show significant improvement in patients' symptoms except for grass pollen injections for hay fever. This could truly be called controversial treatment!

During the last few years companies manufacturing vaccines have succeeded in producing pure extracts which are effective but their increased potency and purity have produced a significant rise in unacceptable side-effects, including anaphylactic death, and some have been withdrawn. The Committee on Safety of Medicines issued (November 1986) a warning to doctors not to use desensitising injections unless they have adequate facilities for resuscitation and they observe the patient for one to two hours after the injection. Most general practitioners have therefore declined to continue this form of treatment. There is also anecdotal evidence that chronic asthmatics may become permanently worse after ill-judged courses of desensitising injections with mixed antigens.

Food desensitisation – can it be done? Desensitising injections of food extracts can work but the effect is short-lived. Some years ago I was involved with Dr Frankland in a trial with twenty patients who were Type I (immediate) sensitive to foods. For example, a man with anaphylactic reactions to wheat arrived in this country from the Far East and found it very difficult to avoid having accidents with wheat contained in foods. He was given a very long course of desensitisation, using between sixty-five and seventy injections with only a minimal increase in concentration on each subsequent injection. The method was carried out by the Rush technique in hospital. This is a dangerous technique and deaths have occurred but full precautions were taken. It was successful in that at the end of the course the man was able to drink beer and eat bread without any problems, but after a month the effect started to decline and he required booster injections. After a while, anaphylactic reactions began to appear to the booster doses so the whole method was abandoned.

Graded normal exposure

This method has a long history, starting with Finkelstein in 1905. It depends on introducing orally a minute dose of the antigen in solution, a dose too small to provoke a reaction, and then step-wise increasing the dose in multiples of about 1.5. It has been used quite frequently to produce tolerance to drugs such as aspirin, paramino-salicylic acid in the treatment of tuberculosis, and penicillin. The desired effect can be achieved within about two weeks but the doses have to be maintained very frequently or the patients rapidly revert to the intolerant state. If a dose of the drug is then given after an interval the anaphylactic reaction reappears. This method has also been tried with inhalation of pollen by hay fever patients. It was found that the incremental dose had to be kept small and the whole process therefore took quite a long time but it could be successful with pollens and moulds which have a seasonal incidence. The effect also appeared to last longer than it did with the drugs but there are no reports of long-term follow-up, so it is very difficult to know whether this method has any long-lasting benefit. It is possible that no desensitisation technique gives permanent cure but merely suppresses the reaction until natural tolerance takes over. In the case of pollens and moulds the antigen is applied through an aerosol by inhalation. The effect may therefore be a mucosal one rather than a systemic one, but as that is the normal portal of entry of the natural antigen this may be effective.

Food desensitization by the oral route. Although this method would have great theoretical advantages and is psychologically more acceptable, it unfortunately does not appear to work very well. Some workers, e.g., Patriarca *et al.* (1979), have reported good results using a method to desensitise one food at a time and have found that by using the slow incremental steps already mentioned it could take up to six months to desensitise to a single food. Others, such as Zanussi (1982), failed to find the method very effective. There are several problems associated with it. Firstly, one can use only one food at a time. Secondly, incremental doses have to be very carefully controlled and accidental ingestion of the food may completely wreck the desensitisation schedule. Thirdly, attempts to speed up the process can result in anaphylactic reactions and, finally, the maximum tolerated dose above which reactions always occur can be too small a dose to be clinically useful.

Neutralising therapy

The scientific basis of neutralisation rests on the observation of the normal inverted U-shaped response curve to increasing doses of allergen. If you incubate the blood of a hay fever sufferer with grass pollen extract in a test tube, too little of the extract has no effect.

As the dose is increased an optimum is reached which provokes maximum histamine release. This dose for grass pollen extract is about one in 10 million.

As the dose is increased still further a point is reached where histamine release is again almost zero.

You can demonstrate this phenomenon using a wide range of doses of grass pollen extract for skin tests. The effect is the same in food allergy and it is often quite easy to demonstrate the same shape of dose-response curve when the whole patient is challenged by eating different doses of food allergen.

The high dose of allergen which produces minimum symptoms is correctly called the masking dose. If used therapeutically it is known as the neutralising dose. Smaller doses than this – 'underdose' – provoke symptoms. Higher doses of allergen may also provoke symptoms, though surprisingly the symptoms of 'overdose' are generally less severe than those of 'underdose'.

When the characteristics of the allergen dose/response curve are investigated by using intradermal injections we find that overdoses produce skin wheals due to histamine release at the site of injection, yet the generalised symptoms, if any, are usually slight. Underdoses often produce generalised symptoms but frequently there is no accompanying local skin response.

Patients who are given regular doses of allergen at the neutralising dose are often protected from illness caused by natural exposure to the same allergen. This appears to be a safe technique and four successful double-blind trials have been published showing that it works with single allergens. In clinical practice the technique appears to be useful and it certainly works better than placebo.

What is less clear, and what has not been shown by objective trials is that making up a mixture of fifty or more antigens by this technique can be equally effective, yet this is common practice.

It should also be noted that neutralisation is a short term effect, not a true 'desensitisation'. The possibility of a sustained effect akin to real desensitisation cannot be ruled out, especially if the dose is repeated frequently over a period of time, but this appears to happen only to a very small percentage of those who first start the treatment.

To many minds, particularly when it was first developed by Rinkel to treat patients, this method has appeared totally illogical. Failure to accept even the easily demonstrated dose-response curve to allergen on skin testing marked the dividing of the ways between the so-called 'conventional allergists' using desensitising injections, and others who have called themselves clinical ecologists. Sadly for their patients there is still little dialogue between the two groups.

In practice the neutralisation technique suffers from several disadvantages. First, determining the neutralising points of a large number of antigens is time-consuming and expensive. Second, the neutralising point for an allergen may not be stable. If it changes the dose of allergen which initially neutralised and protected the patient will start to provoke symptoms instead. As a result many patients require regular re-testing and adjustment of their treatment which is almost as laborious as the initial testing.

The third problem is more subtle. The section of the immune system which controls sensitisation and the manufacture of new antibody is essentially 'silent'. It recognises antigen with its own antibody-like receptors independently of the mechanisms which express allergy. A dose of allergen which is adjusted to neutralise the expression of allergy may at the same time stimulate this 'silent' part of the immune system, ultimately worsening the allergy and favouring the development of new sensitivities. There are many allergy sufferers to whom this seems to have happened. The final problem is that immoderate testing procedures can train patients to react psychologically when they believe they are exposed to allergens to which they are really not sensitive. Some years ago this problem was aired in the correspondence columns of The Lancet.

Pulse steroid therapy

In the early 1950s a chest physician named Houghton tried to treat a number of patients who had violent reactions to food with the newly marketed ACTH (adreno-cortico-trophic-hormone). Some of these reactions, for example, urticaria after eating strawberries, might not have been truly atopic. Houghton's method was to give his patients 120 units of ACTH three times a day for two days. He later added 50 mg of prednisolone as well. On the second day the patients had a full meal of the food containing the suspect allergen and thereafter all treatment was stopped. They then found that they could eat the food which had previously upset them, without being affected by it. These findings were presented to the British Allergy Society but unfortunately were not published. Houghton was alleged to have treated some 200 patients with good results and there seemed to be no significant side-effects from such large doses of steroid over a two-day period. Unfortunately, nobody has followed up this work.

Enzyme potentiated desensitisation (EPD)

This method depends on the ability of the enzyme beta glucuronidase to enhance the sensitising or desensitising effect of antigen which is administered at the same time. The method was first developed about twenty years ago and the initial laboratory work on animals was published between 1972 and 1975 by McEwen *et al*. To increase its safety and produce slow delivery of the antigen, a method of delivery was developed whereby the antigen and betaglucuronidase were applied to the skin over a small scarified area in a plastic cup and absorption was enhanced using hyaluronidase. The scrape, using a sharp blade, is transiently uncomfortable but probably no worse than an intradermal injection. The plastic cup is left *in situ* for twenty-four hours and thereafter the abrasion on the skin heals without scarring. Some patients have received up to sixty doses without any significant local problems. Serious systemic side-effects have not so far been reported. The treatment can also be delivered by intradermal injection, in which case hyaluronidase is not required. When a suitably low and tolerance-inducing dose of antigen is administered by this method, the beta glucuronidase greatly enhances the effect so that clinically useful tolerance is achieved. Compared with other forms of immunotherapy the dose of antigen required is extremely small and multiple antigens can be combined in the same vaccine. If necessary, further improvement in the desensitising effect can be obtained by using nutritional co-factors.

The first double-blind clinical trial in human beings was done in 1967, using grass pollen as the antigen. The vaccine was used to protect against a grass pollen challenge in patients with hay fever provoked during the winter months. More recently, Ortolani (personal communication) treated over 1400 hay fever patients for over four years, using the single injection technique, and compared this method with orthodox desensitising injections. EPD showed complete clearance of symptoms in 13% of patients, against only 5% using conventional injections. 20% of patients with EPD showed no significant improvement, against 15% using conventional treatment; good to moderate responses in the intervening group were approximately the same, but patients having conventional therapy needed 12 injections each year against one dose of EPD, and side-effects were much less using EPD. None of the EPD patients had any generalised reaction, against 5% of those using conventional injections, and localised reactions in the arm were confined to 5% in the EPD group, compared with 15% in the conventional injection group. There would seem to be distinct advantages in using EPD for pollen hyposensitisation.

EPD used to treat patients with ulcerative colitis. To explore the possibility that EPD could be used to treat food allergy a group of patients with ulcerative colitis was treated using a double-blind placebo technique in which conventional drug therapy was not changed. Five doses of EPD or placebo were given over a ten-month period. The placebo used was saline. There were forty-two patients in each group. Patients were assessed by symptoms and by the need for intervention therapy, that is, blood transfusion or colectomy, by an independent team of doctors. After twelve months there was little to choose between the two groups. Improvement in the treated group became obvious after approximately fourteen months from the start of treatment. Subjectively, thirteen of the forty-two patients believed that they were much better, whereas only two in the control group did. Sigmoidoscopy findings over the ensuing fourteen months showed there was one classified as Grade 3 in the treated group and eight in the placebo control group. Three patients in the control group underwent emergency proctocolectomy, but none of those in the treated group did so. The amount of prednisolone used in the placebo group in the second year was considerably greater than the amount used in the treated group, and this included two five-day regime treatments for severe colitis.

Eczema appears to be another condition which lends itself to EPD treatment and isolated examples of improvement in both joint mobility and calcification have been seen in severe rheumatoid arthritis following EPD.

From these examples it will be seen that EPD can be effective treatment for patients with multiple food allergy who have chronic illness of one kind or another. Furthermore, it would appear to be possible to desensitise patients to a number of food allergens, even though the precise diagnosis/identification of these allergens has not been possible beforehand. The treatment is not particularly difficult or expensive, requiring only four or five applications a year. Although the effect may gradually wear off it can be sustained by occasional maintenance therapy. Compared with other forms of treatment, its effectiveness may be less apparent in the short term, and the full effects may not be seen until two years after the start of therapy. Obviously, more scientific work is required to confirm some of these observations but in the meantime this treatment is available for those with complex food intolerance who have found other forms of treatment difficult to maintain.

REFERENCES

Blackley, C. H. (1873, reprinted 1959). *Experimental Researches on the Causes and Nature of Catarrhus Aestivus*, p. 86. (Baillière, Tindall and Cox.)

Finkelstein, H. (1905). Kuhmilch ab Ursache Erhahrumstorungen bei Sauglingen. *Monatsschr. Kinderheilkd.*, **4**, 65–72

Frankland, A. W. and Augustin R. (1954). Prophylaxis of summer hay fever and asthma. Controlled trial comparing crude grass pollen extracts with isolated main pollen component. *Lancet*, **i**, 1055

McEwen, L. M. (1972). Enzyme potentiated hyposensitization I. *Int. Arch. Allergy*, **42**, 152–8

McEwen, L. M. (1973). Enzyme potentiated desensitisation II. *Ann. Allergy*, **31**, 769–83

McEwen, L. M. *et al.* (1973). Enzyme potentiated desensitisation III. *Ann. Allergy*, **31**, 543–50

McEwen, L. M. *et al.* (1975). Enzyme potentiated desensitisation IV. *Ann. Allergy*, **34**, 290–5

McEwen, L. M. (1975). Enzyme potentiated desensitisation V. *Ann. Allergy*, **35**, 98–103

Noon, L. (1911). Prophylactic innoculation against hay fever. *Lancet*, **i,** 1572

Patriarca, G. *et al.* (1979). *Food Allergy*, pp. 131–4. (Massom Italia, Milan)

Rinkel, H. J. *et al.* (1964). The diagnosis of food allergy. *Arch. Otolaryngol.*, **79,** 71

Zanussi, C. (1982). Food allergy treatment. *Clin. Immunol. Allergy*, **2,** 221–40

Appendix 1

Tap-water contaminants and illness caused thereby

A. J. Franklin

Water is essential to all living things and the notion that water could produce allergic disease or any kind of disease seems initially quite preposterous. How could any living thing become intolerant? If we are talking about pure water I would have to agree, but most of us in the Western world take delivery of our drinking and bathing water from a tap connected to a system of water distribution from distant reservoirs. En route, that water may have descended through polluted air to fall on contaminated soil, been extracted from rivers, and circulated through processing plants and areas of human habitation, which add to the pollution. In some cases, having passed through one area of habitation, the sewage which results may be discharged, after some cleaning up, into those same rivers which further downstream are used for the supply of potable water for the next habitable area.

On a recent estimate (Goodman, 1982) there are over 3500 identifiable organic micropollutants present in drinking water supplies and many more in sewage effluents. Only some 25% of the total number were capable of being analysed and although many are naturally occurring compounds the man-made compounds have a tendency to be more persistent in the aquatic environment (Richardson, 1982; Ongerth *et al.*, 1973). There are probably more than 100,000 of these synthetic compounds in common use, as well as physiologically active steroids and sex hormones, particularly in the run-off from land where animals breed. It is not only expensive but technically difficult to clean up potable water, despite legislation. Some countries, e.g., USA and Canada, have proposed limits of $100\,\mu g/l$ and $350\,\mu g/l$ respectively for the content of tri-halo-methanes in water (Goodman, 1982). Chlorination seems to be responsible for most of the toxicity, as chlorine combines with many natural organic compounds found in humic water to produce both volatile and non-volatile compounds. It has been shown that these compounds, especially chloroform, can be found both in serum and urine after drinking water containing them, unlike the case with uncontaminated well water (Reunanen and Kronell, 1982). Chlorine is used to sterilise the

133

water and appears to be the cheapest and most effective way of removing bacteria.

Toxicity

Nitrates

Nitrates in water, derived largely from fertilisers applied to the soil from which water drains into rivers and reservoirs, have been known for many years to cause methaemoglobinaemia, which leads to persistent cyanosis and respiratory distress in infants. Prolonged boiling of water in food preparation may do the same by concentrating the nitrate. (*Community Medicine*, 1972).

Softened water

Many water authorities soften water with soda lime and readjust the pH with carbon dioxide. Domestic softeners use an ion exchange resin charged with common salt. Drinking soft water can cause hypernatraemic dehydration in babies and young children and over a longer period several studies have shown a reverse correlation between hypertension, cardiovascular deaths and water hardness (Crawford *et al.*, 1980; Pocock *et al.*, 1980).

Birth Defects

Nitrates have also been implicated in causing an increase in congenital defects, especially neural tube defects. A study in South Australia (Scrogg, 1982) showed that in the Mount Gambier region, where more than twice the number of malformations than elsewhere was recorded during 1968–76, the underground water supply was high in nitrate levels. These nitrates are known to be converted to N-nitroso compounds in the body, especially in the stomach, intestines and bladder, and they also cross the placental barrier. Experimentally they have been shown to be teratogenic to several species of small mammal, although a further study (Dreosti *et al.*, 1984) failed to demonstrate this effect in an animal model. N-nitroso compounds may also be preformed in foodstuffs and water.

Cancer incidence

Nitrates and N-nitroso compounds have again been implicated in the incidence of gastro-intestinal and bladder cancer (Swann, 1975). An epidemiological study in London in 1981 (Swann, 1975; Beresford, 1981), taken together with some studies in the USA (Beresford, 1983; Alaranja *et al.*, 1978; Page *et al.*, 1976), suggests that stomach and urinary tract cancers are associated with the use of recycled river waters as a source of drinking water. The causes of this effect were not positively identified but it was suggested that complex organic micropollutants present in industrial and domestic sewage effluent might be involved, or chlorine in drinking water (Salg, 1977). The question of whether water nitrates cause cancer remains open but chloroform is certainly suspected. In the USA, fourteen of the thirty-three most frequently found organic contaminants in groundwater were tested for carcinogenicity in animals by the National Cancer Institute. Eleven of the fourteen were carcinogenic in at least one species of animal (Metzler, 1982).

Minerals

Copper, aluminium and lead are known to be toxic to the central nervous system, but calcium and magnesium may be beneficial as they increase the hardness of the water. Zinc concentrations in pregnant women and in newborns seem to depend on the level found in their drinking water. Low zinc levels have been associated with pregnancy toxaemia and intra-uterine growth retardation (Poradorsky, 1984). Selenium is poisonous in large amounts but beneficial in optimum amounts, affording protection against heart disease, arthritis and cancers, especially breast cancer. Very little manganese and iron are found in drinking water (Gillies, 1982). Sodium intake seemed to bear little correlation with blood pressure in a group of English adolescents (Robertson, 1984).

Effect of tap-water on tissue cultures

Tap-water can inhibit the culture of amniotic fluid cell cultures, resulting in their failure 'to take' (Mulcahy, 1983).

Viral contamination

Viruses derived from the use of sludge on the land may contaminate food grown on the land if the food is eaten raw, for up to one year after it has been applied. Rotavirus is a hazard, as it has been shown to survive conventional treating of drinking water, and it can survive for long periods (Sattar et al., 1984).

Effect on immune system

In an experimental mouse model the use of acidified, chlorinated or tetracycline-added water did not significantly alter humoral immune responses or delayed hypersensitivity reactions. There was some reduction in foot pad response to sheep erythrocytes in the mice drinking the tetracycline water, and in the mice drinking acidified water there was a reduction in their ability to clear particulate foreign matter from the blood via macrophages (Hermann et al., 1982).

Allergic reactions

The mechanism of allergic reactions to tap-water contaminants remains obscure, but reactions indistinguishable from reactions to food, inhalants or chemical allergens are frequently found in allergic patients. Rapp (1972) reported two patients who developed angioedema and urticaria after drinking tap-water and the author has seen one girl who developed it after contact, but only on certain days. Allergic reactions to an endotoxin in tap-water obtained from a small lake contaminated with gram-negative bacteria were reported by Minittari *et al.* (1980). Tap-water has been found to cause diarrhoea in the irritable bowel syndrome in ten cases reported by Alun-Jones *et al.* (1983) in Cambridge, England, and hyperactivity in children (see Chapter 8). Radcliffe (personal communication) conducted a single-blind trial using boiled tap-water as placebo in one child with hyperactive behaviour. Wilson (1982, 1983) has recorded the symptoms found in twelve patients with tap-water hypersensitivity, confirmed by challenge tests.

Effects of contaminants

The main effects of tap-water are found on the following systems:
   Skin: eczema, itching, redness, flaking dryness, angioedema, urticaria
   Gastro-intestinal tract: mouth ulcers, dysphagia, abdominal distension, flatulence, chronic diarrhoea
   Central nervous system: headache, insomnia, irritability, tiredness, hyperactive behaviour, feelings of unreality
   Genito-urinary: frequency/urgency of micturition, irritation
   Chest: tightness, cough, thick sputum, asthma
   Joints: stiffness, pain, Raynaud's phenomenon.

Examples

Baby N., aged 4 months, had screamed perpetually for two months, had a bright red exfoliative rash and diarrhoea which persisted despite changing from breast to goats', to soya milk. Antibiotics appeared to exacerbate the condition, which was resistant to topical and systemic steroids. In hospital deionised-distilled water with soya milk abated all symptoms. On return home all the symptoms returned after the first bottle feed and the baby screamed almost non-stop for twenty-four hours and began to exfoliate. On changing from tap-water to bottled mineral (spring) water the baby fell asleep after the first feed. The diarrhoea ceased within twenty-four hours and the skin healed in five days. Three subsequent challenges between 5 and 10 months of age produced immediate relapse. From 1 year onwards he was able to tolerate the tap-water.

Two brothers, aged 5 and 2, presented with uncontrollable diarrhoea – six or seven loose stools per day – and enuresis. On investigation (including jejunal biopsy) neither showed evidence of malabsorption or allergy (skin prick tests and RAST). Dietary exclusion of common foods (milk and wheat) made a marginal improvement. Purified (double-distilled) drinking water in place of tap-water produced immediate improvement, with one normal stool per day and dry beds at night. Both boys were challenged three times, each challenge producing relapse.

A retired man aged 62 complained of abdominal discomfort, having passed three or four soft stools per day for about twenty years. He began to develop extreme muscle weakness and lethargy. Some improvement was obtained by the use of oral prednisolone, 15 mg per day. Exclusion of dairy foods, wheat and coffee produced a rapid return to normal and steroids were discontinued. A single yoghurt portion produced sudden and severe relapse which lasted for three days. On holiday in Austria he was able to eat all 'forbidden' foods without getting symptoms, but on his return to England these returned. When he replaced tap-water with bottled mineral water he recovered and again was able to eat the previously excluded foods.

A 9-year-old girl with life-long eczema gained considerable improvement after excluding dairy foods (milk products and egg). On holiday in the Mediterranean her skin cleared completely and she was again able to eat dairy foods and drink milk. Within forty-eight hours of return to England she relapsed until she obtained an activated carbon filter for both drinking and washing water (Mayrei), when again her skin healed.

A number of ecologists (for example, Morgan, 1976; Randolph, and Ross, 1980 Mackarness, 1980) have testified to the fact that some very sensitive persons react allergically to tap-water. In view of the available knowledge on the contamination of tap-water this ought not to surprise us. A better way of disinfecting water without using chlorine should help to make potable water more tolerable. Meanwhile, a simple home filter using activated charcoal granules can help many sensitive people.

References

Alaranja, M. *et al.* (1978). In Jolley, R. L., Goocher, H. and Hamilton, D. H. Jnr (eds) *Water Chlorination, Environmental Impact and Health Effects*, Vol. 2, pp 395–409. (Ann Arbor, Science, Ann Arbor, MI)

Alun-Jones V. *et al.* (1983). Food intolerance and the irritable bowel. *Lancet*, Sept 10, 633–4

Beresford, S. A. A. (1981). The relationship between water quality and health in the London area. *Int. J. Epidemiol.*, **10**, 103–15

Beresford, S. A. A. (1983). Cancer incidence and reuse of drinking water. *Am. J. Epidemiol.*, **117** (3), 258–68

Community Medicine (1972). **127,** 133. Quoted in Martindale, (1982) *Extra Pharmacopoeia* 28th edn p. 1669

Crawford, M. D. *et al.* (1980). Studies on the relationship between cardiovascular disease and the softness of water. 1971. *Lancet*, **2**, 327

Dreosti, I. E. *et al.* (1984). Mount Gambier drinking water and birth defects. *Med. J. Aust.*, **141,** 409–11

Gillies, M. E. (1982). Estimates of daily mineral intakes from drinking water. *Human Nutr. Appl. Nutr.*, **36A,** 287–92

Goodman, A. H. (1982). Control of organic micropollutants in relation to public health. Conference Report *Organic Micropollutants in Water*, p 79. Institute of Biology, London

Hermann, L. M. *et al.* (1982). Prolonged response to acid, chlorine or tetracycline in the drinking water. Effects of delayed-type hypersensitivity, haemaglutination titres and reticulo endothelial clearance rates in mice. *Lab. Animal Sci.* **32,** 603–8

Mackarness, R. (1980). In *Chemical Victims*, p 137. (London: Pan Books)

Metzler, D. F. (1982). Health implications of organics in groundwater. *Am. J. Pub. Health* **72,** 1323–4

Minittari, A. *et al.* (1980). Letter in *Lancet*, **2,** 89

Morgan, J. T. (1976). The water problem. In Dickey, L. D. *Clinical Ecology*, pp 306–9. (Thomas, Illinois)

Mulcahy, M. T. (1983). The hazards of tap water. Letter in *Pre-natal diagnosis*, **3,** 81

Ongerth, H. J. *et al.* (1973). Public health aspects of organics in water. *J. Am. Waterworks Assoc.*, **65**, 495–8

Page, T. *et al.* (1976). Drinking water and cancer mortality in Louisiana. *Science*, **193**, 55–7

Pocock, S. J. *et al.* (1980). British regional heart study: a significant negative association between water hardness and cardiovascular mortality. *Br. Med. J.*, **280**, 1243

Poradovsky, K. (1984). Zinc in vital environment and its relationship to human reproduction. *Cesk. Gynackol.*, **49**, 243–7

Randolph, T. G. and Moss, R. W. (1980). The water supply. In *An Alternative Approach to Allergies*, pp 62–3. (New York: Lippincott and Crowell)

Rapp, D. J. (1972). Letter in *J. Am. Med. Assoc.*, **221**, 305

Reunanen, M. and Kronell, R. (1982). Determination of volatile hydrocarbons in raw and drinking water, human serum and urine by Electron Capture G.C. *J. Chromatograph. Sci.*, **20**, 449–54

Richardson, M. (1982). Discussion. In Conference Report *Organic Micropollutants in Water*, p 81. (London: Institute of Biology)

Robertson, J. S. (1984). Water sodium, urinary electrolytes and blood pressure of adolescents. *J. Epidemiol. Comm. Health*, **38**, 186–94

Salg, J. (1977). Cancer mortality – rates and drinking water quality in the Ohio River Valley. Doctoral thesis. University of North Carolina, Chapel Hill

Sattar, S. A. *et al.* (1984). Rotavirus survival in conventionally treated drinking water. *Can. J. Microbiol.*, **30**, 653–6

Scrogg, R. K. (1982). Birth defects and household water supply. *Med. J. Aust.*, **2**, 577–9

Swann, P. F. (1975). The toxicology of nitrate, nitrite and N-nitroso compounds. *J. Sci. Food. Agric.*, **26**, 1766–70

Wilson, C. W. M. (1982). Hypersensitivity to mains tap water in adults, its clinical features and treatment. *Nutr. Health*, **1**, 85–91

Wilson, C. W. M. (1983). Hypersensitivity to mains tap water in children, its clinical features and treatment. *Nutr. Health*, **2**, 51–63

Appendix 2

The role of free radicals in health and disease

B. Halliwell

Editor's note: The following brief summary is included partly because of its intrinsic interest and also partly for the benefit of those who may believe that all food supplied to allergic people should be totally free from additives of all kinds. The subject may become of practical importance in the future if food marketed has been sterilised by the use of ionising radiation.

The concept of a group of highly reactive substances participitating in biological activity and equal to the activity of histamines and prostaglandins has been known to chemists for some years. These substances are known as free radicals. Free radicals are any species of chemical containing one or more unpaired electrons. They may play an important part in a number of clinical conditions, such as rheumatoid arthritis, the respiratory distress syndrome of the newborn and the action of a number of pharmaceutical agents. One of the most common of these free radicals is known as the hydroxyl radical; it is produced when water is exposed to ionising radiation. Normally the larger volume of water is able to absorb the hydroxyl radicals so that their activity is diminished, but they will attack any molecule within a living organism. They have a particular predilection for proteins and membrane lipids. Such interaction may actually, and usually does, provoke a chain reaction in which further free radicals are produced. For example, when the membrane lipids are attacked by hydroxyl radicals, lipid radicals and lipid peroxides are formed. These, in turn, produce peroxy radicals, which can react to produce further lipid radicals and so on *ad infinitum* as long as there is any substrate left to be attacked. This may explain why ionising radiation damage can go on for a long time after the initial exposure. Lipid peroxides can decompose to form cytotoxic products which, even in minute quantities, have an activity comparable to that of prostaglandins and leucotriene intermediates and may be involved in both inflammation and cell division.

If food is irradiated for sterilisation purposes it may start off a process of lipid peroxidation as described above. In order to counteract and stop this process antioxidants such as BHA, BHT and vitamin E are added to the food and these interfere with the peroxy radical and so stop the chain reaction. Unfortunately, in some sensitive subjects the antioxidants themselves and less reactive oxidases formed from them may also have clinical effects which are undesirable.

Oxygen may behave like a free radical, particularly if it comes in contact with anaerobic processes. Aerobic tissues have learned to develop their own antioxidants, but increasing the concentration of oxygen leads more readily to free radical activity and tissue damage, as, for example, in the neonatal condition known as retrolental fibroplasia. This kind of damage can be amelioriated by adequate vitamin E availability. 5% of oxygen gas contains another very much more active free radical known as superoxide and the proportion increases with increased concentrations of oxygen. Superoxide radicals can be modified by the enzyme superoxide dismutase and converted to hydrogen peroxide. This in turn can be eliminated by glutathione peroxidase, which requires the presence of selenium ions.

Not all free radicals are bad, however. They are very useful in the phagocytic cells of the body when they are ingesting invading bacteria. Superoxide is formed at the point on the cell membrane where the particle is ingested and assists in killing the bacteria. In chronic granulomatous disease there is a deficiency in the production of superoxide by the neutrophil and neutrophils therefore use superoxide to kill bacteria. If the production of neutrophils is overactive for any reason, sometimes an excess of superoxide is produced and this may increase tissue damage. This is particularly so in chronic illnesses such as rheumatoid arthritis, where the phagocytes themselves may damage tissues through interference with arachidonic metabolism. Some of the side-effects of drugs might be caused by free radicals: for example, the cardiomyopathy associated with adriamycin and the lung damage associated with paraquat inhalation.

Free radical activity can be increased in the presence of iron, particularly low molecular weight iron. Other metals by themselves seem to have no effect, but aluminium in combination with iron may enhance the activity, as in dialysis encephalopathy. Tissue damage itself increases the availability of free radicals and also low molecular weight iron and therefore may become a self-perpetuating condition. Damage to the brain, either toxic or some other, is particularly well able to promote free radical reactions. The brain cells contain a lot of polyunsaturated fatty acids and iron and cerebrospinal fluid has few antioxidants to counteract the free radical reactions.

It is certainly possible to estimate free radical activity in foodstuffs and it may become important to do so in the future. It may be useful to recognise the role of antioxidants when one is considering tissue damage which may result from allergic inflammatory reactions.

Appendix 3

Definitions

Allergy From two Greek words, *allos* (other) and *ergon* (work). It was originally used by Von Pirquet to describe a change in the body's reaction to an antitoxin, which usually occurs after two or more exposures to it. This is important because initial exposure, which, if it produces a later reaction, may be called sensitisation, does not produce any noticeable effect. This is the basis of immunisation. More recently immunologists have tried to confine the definition to reactions which stimulate the production of specific IgE antibody in the blood.

Allergen Any substance (usually harmless) which induces and provokes an allergic response.

Anaphylaxis A severe and sometimes fatal immediate response to challenge from an antigen which affects several bodily systems simultaneously, leading to vascular collapse (hypotensive shock) and acute breathlessness.

Antibody A blood protein produced in response to the introduction of a foreign substance which penetrates the intact organism.

Antigen A substance that can produce a specific antibody.

Atopy From the Greek word *atopos* (atypical or unusual). Used (by Coca in 1935) to describe the state of an individual who has an hereditary tendency to produce immediate hypersensitivity following allergen challenge leading to the production of IgE antibody. It usually relates to specific disease states such as asthma, rhinitis, eczema and urticaria. It may be identified clinically by the demonstration of a positive skin prick test to one or more antigens.

Basophils White blood cells capable of releasing mediator chemicals in the blood in response to antigen challenge.

Complement A generic term for a group of blood proteins which are often involved, sometimes in sequence, in inflammatory and other reactions. They interact with immune proteins and blood cells such as leucocytes and platelets, leading to the release of chemical mediators such as histamine. They have many different functions, but when combined with antigen/antibody complexes they become inactive or 'fixed'.

Degranulation The breakdown of storage granules in basophils and mast cells to release their component chemical mediators.

Eosinophils   White blood cells associated with allergic inflammation or parasitic inflammation. The presence of a high circulating eosinophilia would suggest an allergic or parasitised state.

Hapten   A small chemical molecule capable of being bound to a protein to form an allergen.

Hypersensitivity   A state of readiness in which the immune system can respond either rapidly (immediate hypersensitivity) by the release of chemicals causing inflammation and smooth muscle contraction (e.g. histamine), or slowly (delayed or cell-mediated hypersensitivity) by the mobilisation of T-lymphocytes which produce a more gradual and sustained inflammatory response involving invasion of white blood cells to the site where the antigen has lodged.

Immune/Immunity   A defence system of the body, based on the lymphatic system and its circulating lymphocytes, capable of mounting an offensive against invading foreign protein or organisms. It includes the spleen, thymus, tonsil and lymphatic glands, as well as the blood cells. The gut is particularly well endowed with additional structures: Peyer's patches, appendix, caecal and colonic patches for the GALT – Gut associated lymphoid tissue system. The latter is involved in the control of the entry of food proteins.

Immune complexes   A combination of antigen with one or more specific antibodies capable of fixing complement and leading to inflammation.

Immunoglobulins   A class of blood proteins associated with immune function. IgA is also found in secretions, especially of the respiratory and gastro-intestinal tracts. IgG antibodies are formed first in response to antigens and quantitatively probably represent exposure to the appropriate antigens. There are at least four subclasses recognised. Deficiency is associated with recurrent and uncontrolled infection. IgM is a large molecular weight antibody formed in the wall of the gut, IgE is associated with atopy and the role of IgD is still being explored. Infants are particularly deficient in Ig's, reaching their peak low level (between maternal passive transfer and infant's own production developing) at about 3 months of age.

Inflammation   Classically a triple response to injury, consisting of redness, heat and swelling which frequently causes pain, brought about by neurological, vascular and cellular infiltrative activity at the local site.

Intolerance/Tolerance   Food intolerance is the preferred term for any abnormal response to food. It can be due to immunological, toxic or other non-immunological causes. Tolerance here refers to a state of specific unresponsiveness to an antigen following repeated exposure to it.

Leucotrienes   Specific chemical substances (mediators) released following the degranulation of mast cells or basophils. Previously known as the slow reacting substance of anaphylaxis – SRS-A.

Lymphocytes   White blood cells produced in the bone marrow, capable of differentiation into T and B cells. The former differentiate further into effector (or killer) cells, helper and suppressor T cells which enhance or suppress the action of the effector cells in eliminating foreign protein by bringing about its destruction. The B cells form the immunoglobulins in response to contact with antigen presented by macrophages.

Macrophages   Amoeboid white blood cells which 'scavenge' the blood and tissues, engulfing foreign protein and antigens and destroying them by direct enzyme action or through contact with the lymphocytes.

Mast cells From the German word *mast* (fattened seed). They are special mucosal cells which appear to be stuffed full of granules – chemical packages capable of being released into surrounding tissues when the cell membrane is activated by the linking of two or more antibody receptor sites on the cell surface by an appropriate antigen. These chemicals, e.g., histamine, platelet activating factor and leucotrienes, represent the chemical mediators of the allergic response leading to the secondary inflammatory (cellular) response.

Pathogenic Causing disease.

Prostaglandins A group of chemical hormones found in many tissues of the body. They are often found in association with immune mediator reactions.

RAST The radio-allergosorbent test, a test to measure the amount of specific IgE in the blood.

Receptor sites Areas on the surface of lymphocytes, mast cells and others, shaped to fit exactly specific antigens, thereby generating an ionic response which triggers mediator chemical release.

Appendix 4

Further reading

Scientific

1. Brostoff, J. and Challacombe, S. J. *et seq.* (1987). *Food Allergy and Intolerance*, p 1016. Baillière Tindall
2. Brostoff, J. and Challacombe, S. J. (1982). Food allergy. *Clin. Immunol. Allergy*, **2** (1), 255
3. Lessof, M. (1983). *Clinical Reactions to Food*, p 215. J. Wiley & Sons
4. The First and Second Fisons Food Allergy Workshops (1980 and 1983). The Medicine Publishing Foundation, Oxford
5. Scowen, P. and Medhurst, G. (1985). *Food Allergy*, p 93. B. Edsall & Co., London
6. Gerrard, J. W. (1980). *Food Allergy*. C. C. Thomas, Springfield, Illinois
7. Francis, D. (1987). *Diets for Sick Children*, 4th edn. Blackwell Scientific Publishers, Oxford, London and Edinburgh

Popular

1. Minchin, M. (1986). *Food for Thought*, p 263. Unwin (Australian edn); Oxford University Press (British edn)
2. Eagle, R. (1979). *Eating and Allergy*. Futura Books
3. Armstrong, D. and Cant, A. (1986) *The Allergy-free Cookbook*. Octopus Books, London
4. Rapp, D. (1980). *Allergies and Your Family*, p 327. Sterling Publishing Co.
5. Rapp, D. (1979). *Allergies and the Hyperactive Child*. Simon and Schuster, New York
6. Lewis, S. (1986). *Allergy? Think about Food*, 2nd edn. Wisebuy Publications, London
7. Mackarness, R. (1978). *Not All in the Mind*. Pan Books
8. Mackarness, R. (1980). *Chemical Victims*. Pan Books
9. Morrow-Brown, H. (1985). *The Allergy and Asthma Reference Book*. Harper & Row

10. Workman, E., Hunter, J. and Alun-Jones, V. (1984). *The Allergy Diet*. Methuen
11. Polunin, M. (1984). *The Right Way to Eat*. J. M. Dent & Sons
12. Templeton, L. (1984). *The Right Food for Your Kids*. Century, London
13. Mansfield, P. and Munro, J. (1987). *Chemical Children*. Century, London

Appendix 5

Example of an elimination diet

Diet free from artificial food additives (i.e. Preservatives, Colours, & Flavours) and Dairy foods

In order to eliminate these food additives, it is necessary to base the diet on fresh foods eliminating all but permitted manufactured foods.

It is also necessary to eliminate non-food sources of these additives e.g. toothpaste, pastilles, lozenges and medicines. Your doctor should be consulted about these if you are unsure.

CAREFUL EXAMINATION OF LABELS will show if the manufactured food contains artificial preservative, colour, or flavour. Any food which states that it is free from artificial additives may be eaten, provided that it is also free of dairy foods, which this diet must also avoid.

IF THERE IS EVER ANY DOUBT ABOUT A PRODUCT – AVOID IT.

FOODS ALLOWED	*FOODS FORBIDDEN*
Fresh meat, poultry and offal. White fish.	Luncheon meats, salami, sausages, beefburgers, paté, black pudding etc. Ham, bacon, all barbecued types of chicken. Frozen fish with coloured coating, fish fingers. No smoked products, as artificial colours may be used to enhance the colour obtained by smoking.

Milk substitute
  Formula S (Cow & Gate) ⎤
  Prosobee (Mead Johnson) ⎬ Soya
  Wysoy (Wyeths) ⎦
  Nutramigen ⎤ (Mead Johnson)
  Pregestimil ⎦
  Goat's milk
	Milk – fresh, skimmed, evaporated, condensed. Coffee-Mate, cream.

147

Vitaquell margarine. Dripping, pure cooking oils and fats.	Butter, other magarines. Cheese, yoghurt, ice-cream. Eggs.
Fresh fruit – lemons, grapefruit, pears, pineapple, melon, avocado, fresh rhubarb.	Almonds, apples, apricots, blackberries, bilberries, gooseberries, raspberries, strawberries, cherries, currants, grapes and raisins, or any products made from grapes (e.g. wine, wine vinegar, jellies) nectarines, oranges, peaches, bananas.
Vegetables – all fresh varieties except those opposite.	Tomatoes and all tomato products. Cucumbers. Instant mashed potato.
Wholemeal bread and flour. Rice, sago, semolina, cornflour. Oatmeal, rolled oats. Kellogg's Cornflakes (malt flavour). Shredded Wheat.	ALL breakfast cereals with colouring and flavouring. White flour and bread. ALL manufactured cakes, biscuits, pastry, doughnuts, etc.
Pure grapefruit or pineapple juice. Homemade lemonade. Cocoa. '7-UP'.	Tea, coffee. ALL carbonated drinks except '7-UP'. Diet drinks, instant mix drinks. Fruit squashes.
Salt, pepper, white vinegar, pure herbs and spices.	Cider and wine vinegar. Monosodium glutamate.
Sugars, syrup, treacle. Pure honey. Homemade or shop jam with permitted fruits and free from additives e.g. Elsenham or Tiptree. Marmite	Bovril.
Homemade sweets (see recipes). Golden Wonder plain crisps.	ALL 'shop bought' sweets and chocolate. Flavoured potato crisps.
Homemade ice-lollies, made with permitted fruit juice. Jellies made with permitted fruit juice, and set with gelatin.	*Miscellaneous* Flavoured puddings, frozen baked goods. Most packet mixes – i.e. soups, cakes, puddings. ALL gravy mixes/cubes. Mint sauces, and flavours. Soy sauce. Prepared mustard.

Sundry Items
Aspirin, Alka Seltzer, coloured vitamins.
ALL toothpastes and tooth powders.
ALL cough drops, and throat lozenges.
Perfumes, coloured and scented soaps.
Bubble bath.

REMINDER – CHECK ALL LABELS VERY CAREFULLY

NOTES

1. Salt may be used for cleaning teeth.
2. Neutrogena or Simple Soap, are unscented and colour free soaps.
3. The fruits and vegetables listed under FOODS FORBIDDEN contain natural SALICYLIC ACID, bananas contain natural BENZOIC ACID. Both of these substances have to be eliminated from the diet. REMOVE all fruits and vegetables listed. If there is a good response to the diet, introduce them back into the diet one at a time. If no reaction occurs leave that item in the diet.
4. VITAQUELL margarine is available in health food shops.
5. The milk substitutes listed may not be suitable for everyone – check with your doctor about this. If no milk substitute is used, a calcium supplement should be prescribed by your doctor.

SAMPLE MENU

BREAKFAST	Grapefruit or pineapple juice. Porridge, or permitted cereal with milk substitute and sugar. Wholemeal bread with Vitaquell margarine. Pure honey, marmite or permitted jam.
MID-MORNING	Milk substitute or permitted fruit juice. Permitted fruit or crisps.
LUNCH	Fresh meat, white fish or poultry. Potatoes, boiled, mashed, chipped or roast. Permitted fresh vegetables or salad. Milk pudding (made with substitute), or permitted fruit.
MID-AFTERNOON	Permitted fruit juice or homemade lemonade. Permitted fruit, or homemade cake or biscuit.

EVENING MEAL   Fresh meat, white fish or poultry.
                                Potatoes or wholemeal bread.
                                Permitted fresh vegetables or salad.
                                Pudding as at lunch, or homemade cake,
                                or permitted fruit.
BED-TIME   Milk substitute, or permitted fruit juice.

RECIPES

OAT BISCUITS   makes 36 small biscuits.
2 oz golden syrup   3 oz rolled oats
1 tbsp water $\frac{1}{2}$ level tsp bicarbonate of soda
2 tbsp pure cooking oil   2 oz wholemeal flour
3 oz sugar   Pinch of salt

Warm the syrup and water together, add the oil. Add to the dry ingredients
and mix well. It should be a dropping consistency. Form into balls, flatten,
and place 2 ins. apart on oiled baking trays. Bake until delicately brown,
350°F, Gas 3–4, for 15–20 minutes. Cool, then store in an airtight tin.

WHOLEMEAL SCONES   Makes 16 scones.
8 oz wholemeal S.R. flour   A little milk substitute
4 oz Vitaquell margarine   Pinch of salt

Mix the flour and salt together, rub in the margarine. Add enough liquid to
bind the mixture. Have a greased and floured baking tin ready. Shape 16
scones and place on the tin. Bake in a hot oven for about 15 minutes.

COOKIES
$1\frac{1}{4}$ oz Vitaquell margarine   1 oz rolled oats or ground rice
$1\frac{1}{2}$ oz sugar $\frac{1}{2}$ tsp cocoa
$\frac{1}{2}$ tsp honey or golden syrup $\frac{1}{4}$ tsp bicarbonate of soda
2 oz wholemeal flour   2 tsp boiling water
Pinch of salt

Melt the margarine, syrup and sugar. Add the dry ingredients. Mix well
adding more water if needed. Form into small balls, place on greaseproof
paper. Flatten slightly. Bake for 15 minutes, 350°F, Gas 4.

VIENNESE WHIRLS
3 oz Vitaquell margarine   3 oz cornflour
1 oz icing sugar

Cream the margarine and sugar. Gradually mix in the flour to make a stiff,
smooth mixture. Roll into small walnut-size balls, and place onto a greased
baking sheet. Flatten with a fork or the back of a spoon. Bake at 400°F, Gas
5, for 8–10 minutes. Cool and dust with a little icing sugar.
Alternatively a little water may be added, and the mixture piped into stars or
bars onto the baking sheet, and baked as above. Join together with a 'butter'
icing made with Vitaquell margarine and icing sugar.

FLAPJACKS

8 oz rolled oats

1 oz sugar

2 tbsp golden syrup

4 oz Vitaquell margarine

Beat the fat and sugar to a cream. Stir in the syrup and oats. Spread evenly in a greased baking tin. Bake in a moderate oven, 350°F, Gas 4, for 30–40 minutes. Cut into squares, but leave in the tin until cold, as they are rather fragile.

NUTTIES

4 oz Vitaquell margarine

1 oz golden syrup

4 oz sugar

7 oz rolled oats

$\frac{1}{2}$ level tsp salt

2 oz chopped walnuts or peanuts

Melt the fat and syrup together, but do not allow to become too hot. Mix the other ingredients together, pour in the melted mixture, and combine well to make a crumbly mixture. Spread in a flat, greased baking tin, smoothing the top with a knife. Cook very slowly until lightly browned, 350°F, Gas 4, for 30–45 minutes. Mark in fingers and leave in the tin until almost cold.

CARAMEL TOFFEE

12 oz granulated sugar

$3\frac{1}{2}$ oz Vitaquell margarine

$\frac{1}{4}$ cup of milk substitute or water

$\frac{1}{4}$ cup of golden syrup

Mix all the ingredients together, and bring to the boil over a low heat. Boil for approx. 25–30 minutes, or until the mixture will set when tested in cold water. Pour into a flat tray, and mark into squares.

NOTE

Any 'homemade' recipes may be used, provided that all the ingredients are permitted.

Postscript

Living and coping with allergy – a parent's view

J. Thorn

To many people the diagnosis of allergy or food intolerance comes as no great surprise, usually because they have already spent quite some time coming to terms with it before ever having consulted a doctor. If you find yourself continually in distress after having eaten a particular food or having been in contact with a particular substance, you are hardly likely to carry on using it; it's usually at the stage of desperation that professional help is sought. In some cases it is not easy to recognise the problem straight away and if the affected person happens to be a child the desperation is more acute. Parents may consider themselves fortunate to have met with an open minded and sympathetic doctor who has managed to get their problem looked at more thoroughly. The final diagnosis usually comes with a sense of relief – confirmation that there is definitely something not quite in order. As the subject can be so controversial, the diagnosis serves as a public pronouncement that you have not had the equivalent of a brainstorm. A sense of foreboding often ensues; how is this declaration going to affect everyone's lives? What is the treatment?

The doctor's final diagnosis may just mean little more than a modification of an established lifestyle. The main areas needing to be covered are good backup support and additional nutritional guidance; this sometimes can be found in your local area, but all too often the help of the various support groups is vital at this stage. But for those so diagnosed with no prior knowledge of the condition, this time can be a nightmare! They feel on the one hand a sense of relief that somebody is doing something positive about their problem, but on the other hand their lives have immediately been thrown into turmoil and they are desperately in need of good counselling; the doctors have a limited amount of time that they can give the patient.

Some people might be gifted with analytical minds but the majority are thrown into confusion and despair on learning not only that eating and domestic shopping habits have to be changed but also family budgetting is going to be sorely taxed; this is not going to be for the short term but for an indefinite period with no hope, for the majority, of any financial assistance.

Despite the extreme odds, many soldier on; the slow but sure road to recovery is enough evidence in itself to make the sacrifices worthwhile.

It would be impossible to include a satisfactory detailed guide plan to help every sufferer over every pitfall that they might encounter, or one that could take into consideration every problem encountered on the road to recovery; although each person has certain similarities in their allergy, each case is unique. There are however a number of useful tips that can be passed on from one fellow sufferer to the next, and this can be done through the support groups. These groups help you to keep up with major developments as well as giving you moral support. Developing a flexible attitude is an absolute essential if you are ever going to survive the course.

The 24 hour survival guide

It is always wise to check with your consultant before administering any kind of treatment, no matter how benign it might appear at the time. After a while you will find yourself being quite competent at dealing with a crisis, developing a sixth sense when something is not quite running true to form.

Gastrointestinal

Become adept at making both broth and gruel; for this you need to have a list made up of possible ingredients allowed within the diet. Experiment with these ingredients on yourself first, if your child is a fussy eater, it's better than ending up with a disaster when the time comes. Broth and gruel are an absolute godsend when the child is off his food and you're worried about how to get liquid and nutrients into him. Make the mixtures as varied and as interesting as possible. Suitable preparations to restore the balance of an upset digestive system are BIOBALM, SLIPPERY ELM, COMFREY TEA (well diluted for young children). These are available at health shops. Do always check thoroughly all ingredients, as some could cause problems for particularly sensitive individuals.

Also a small amount of cold pressed olive oil (unrefined) can help those suffering from sensitivity to acidic foods.

A small amount of natural salt or bicarbonate of soda can offset irritant effects of some fruits.

Skin

There is a natural vitamin E cream on the market which is based on avocado and apricot oils, with a non perfumed base. This is useful for surface abrasions. Calendula ointment is also available, suitable for minor burns, skin abrasions and small cuts. Magnesium sulphate is available at chemists; this is useful if dirt has got into the wound and I've even used it to help ease out a deep-seated splinter. A bottle of witch hazel is useful to have in your first aid kit.

Respiratory

There are a number of suitable preparations which can act as 'Rubs' or can be used in the oldfashioned way as an inhalant. Eucalyptus oil is a very economical decongestant, available at local chemists. A small amount of honey and lemon in cooled boiled water is a great asset for a tickly cough, although older people might benefit from having it as hot as they can stand it. Again there are a number of herbal remedies available, but do check on ingredients. Raised temperature, in many instances, can be brought quickly under control by bathing sides of neck, wrists with tepid water; follow up with gentle sponging of other parts of the body that are overheating, making sure that the forehead is left till general temperature has been brought under control, as too rapid cooling can bring on a state of shock.

Action such as this can often eliminate a crisis, but do contact a doctor if symptoms persist.

Behaviour

If angry or over excited the sponging down technique (as for temperature control) works wonders, so you might all get a little wet!

Be prepared to snuggle down with young children, they can often show signs of bad behaviour when they are over tired, and a close snuggle even in an armchair can encourage body rest, even if the child does not seem compliant at first. Use a good book or a favourite toy to make up stories about. With the aid of distraction and the security of being with you, it might even turn out to be one of the high spots of your day!

Keep an observation chart on good times and bad times, then try to predict and prepare for the bad spells; after all, forewarned is forearmed. Try to modify situations that can aggravate, until such times as they are more emotionally able to cope with them. Don't overtire the child unless it can't possibly be avoided. Don't intentionally overexcite. Keep the room at a temperature that the child feels comfortable in; adults are more able to cope with changes in temperature.

Make sure that there is ample time spent away from bright lights. Dark curtains for the bedroom are often a good idea if the child has difficulty getting off to sleep. Even bright colours can disturb some extra sensitive individuals.

Prolonged bouts of bad behaviour, as in adverse reactions, withdrawal symptoms and emotional disturbance, can best be coped with by finding a quiet cool area in which to unwind gradually, with minimum risk to themselves or others, preferably where they are in sight and sound of somebody who cares, so that they do not feel ostracized. Try to let the mood burn out naturally; children often have to be helped to come to terms with themselves. Have a few things around that are particular favourites. Be available, but not hovering; often they are very conscious of the way they have behaved after the event. The child himself will let you know when you are needed. If you take it in your stride the child will soon learn to adapt and will often seek out this spot in the future.

Be prepared to see that it might not necessarily be the child at fault, parents have bad days too!

Try to assess whether the bad behaviour is in any way related to frustration. The mind can often work at a different pace to physical ability. Even mild sight and hearing difficulties can often give rise to frustration and confusion, let alone communication problems within the family and other social situations. Is coordination good? Can the child come to terms with reality and imagination?

Be very positive in praise. Do not ignore unacceptable behaviour; this is often a child's way of testing you. They often feel more secure if they know the acceptable boundaries. Make quite sure that the child understands that it is the behaviour that is unacceptable not the child; a tough exterior does not always cover a tough personality.

Make a list of easy steps towards a goal e.g. sharing the clearing up without making a fuss (then they can't feel the only ones picked on); make sure that each step is recognised and approved. Visible reassurance is vital to many of these children, as emotional development can often be seriously impaired.

Avoid conflict by making sure that there is an agreed set of unwritten rules which must be adhered to; this is for everyone's mutual benefit. Let the child see that you stick by the rules as well, that they are not just for them, even if it means that you have to accept chastisement.

At bedtime try wrapping a fractious infant in an item of your own clothing, or let him cuddle up with it; this often helps to calm him down.

In the case of negativism be firm, constant and rational; have clear rules and explain the choices. Often negativism is used as moral blackmail in order to shift the responsibility for emotional immaturity. Having a firmly structured response helps them to come to terms with this.

Where there are violent outbursts you should remove as quickly as possible any item that can cause injury. Do not inflame situations by getting angry yourself; this only adds fuel to the fire. Try the cooling down technique; this might even turn into a water fight with nobody really getting seriously hurt.

Redirect anger i.e. teddy bashing, paper tearing; this can be turned into positive action when the crisis has abated (teddy hospital, paper fight).

Be prepared to accept that if a child cries constantly through the night it's a sure sign that something is wrong. Be prepared to give up your privacy and peace; after all, this is what parenthood is all about, caring. The child will feel more happy and secure knowing that you care, and will feel more inclined to go it alone, once he gets older, when the discomfort has gone, and as he becomes more independent and peer opinion has its influence. It might seem an age to you, but it is only a small part of a child's life.

No matter what they do make children realize that to you they are special – self esteem is needed for anybody to hold their head up high.

Hyperactivity and food sensitivity

Space out activities – QUIET – ACTIVE, and be aware that despite their apparent inexhaustibility children can often be even more active when they are overtired.

Allow ample time before bedtime for a child to unwind, a time for quiet calm activities in a quiet spot in the house if at all possible. Bedtimes vary enormously so don't assume that because Jimmy next door goes to bed at 8.00 p.m. that is necessarily the time for little Jenny.

Children can have irritatingly long memories, so make sure that the day ends with all differences resolved; a bad night can herald an exhausting day. Moods can be extreme. Make sure *you* take the opportunity to unwind and relax, no matter what time of day it is, so that you can cope with them. Be prepared for maturity in behaviour to show great fluctuations. Steer, rather than direct, cajole, rather than persuade, suggest, rather than tell, prepare, rather than inform.

Give them plenty of time to circumnavigate and come to terms with new situations. They will often say the opposite to what they really mean and expect you to understand this.

They may be very possessive, so make sure that the items to be shared are clearly defined. Make sure that they adapt to separation in small easy stages, with plenty of reassurance: let them have a preview of the places you disappear to, if at all possible, so that you can talk about it afterwards and they don't feel so left out.

Make a special area at home that can be their own private spot. After all life is a long series of adaptations, e.g. family and school, and they need a space to come to terms with this and themselves; they also need a place where they feel secure.

Redirect aggression caused by frustration into positive games where they can develop a feeling of success. Redirect abusive language into creative language; after all, the urge to vocalise is a sign of the need for expression!

Use co-operative moments at home to develop the weaker skills. Often bad behaviour comes from a feeling of inadequacy.

If they are sensitive to colouring pigments avoid the use of crayons, finger paints, coloured play dough, touching glues and coloured tissue paper.

Diet

A lot of emphasis is put on diet, but apart from one or two guide lists and useful recipe books, once you know what you are up against there is very little anybody can do until you get 'stuck in', then the fun and confusion really starts. Here are a few useful tips to stop you really going 'batty' and give you and your family a better chance to come through this metamorphosis in one piece.

Do make a list of permitted foods, leave space to add additional extras, because believe it or not you do find more as you go along. Stick this up somewhere in full view in the kitchen.

Do go out and select some useful books on selective diets; wholefood, vegan and vegetarian cookery. When you are more confident, there are books on macrobiotic cooking, seaweed, pulses and beans.

Don't get obsessed by any one approach; find the recipes that suit your needs and apply them.

Don't rush into all this too quickly or you will have a rebellion on your hands.

Do try to adapt old family favourites to the new ingredients.

Do be cost effective; after all what is the good of making a super meal if you can only afford it once in a blue moon!

Do work your meals around seasonal varieties of fruit and vegetables as this can often be cheaper. Cultivate friendships with keen gardeners and offer to buy produce from them; this can often work out much cheaper, and you are going to need every saving you can make.

Get to know your pulses, grains, nuts etc. slowly – if you rush into things too quickly you won't find the full range of applications, and you can often end up with a disaster, that not only drives you nuts but ruins your chances of persuading the rest of the family that they really are onto a good thing.

Inventiveness is the key, so invent your own names for the concoctions. This usually goes down very well with the children and finally convinces your husband that you're gone right round the bend, therefore he'd better humour you, otherwise there's no knowing what you will do next!

You can have a 'What's For Dinner Game', who can think of the best name? Your valiant efforts can take on a new lease of life when they become known by such names as:

SWEET AND EAT IT – MUM'S SURPRISE – SLIPPERY SLOP — CRISPY CRUSH

Offset your costing by a firm stand at your local health shop, to supply particular items you use a lot of in bulk. If you try to deal with the wholesaler direct you have postage and packing to contend with. However, as a last resort you can deal direct with wholesale, *if* you can make up a reasonably large order – perhaps with a few people grouped together.

If your local supermarket is not supplying the range of goods available from others in the chain, write to the central office.

Seek out the unfamiliar foods in ethnic minority shops – people there will often give you hints on how to use items, and what you do after that is entirely up to you!

Experiment with different textures while cooking i.e. chewy, crunchy, soft or crumbly.

Get the children on your side, 'Johnny chose the meal today, it's his favourite lentil shepherd's pie.'

Sweets – avoid where possible – use as a special treat only, and they should preferably be homemade. 'Carnation' provides a low fat evaporated milk which some are well able to tolerate, and it is useful in making such things as old fashioned toffee.

Children often do better on four small meals a day, so invent special nutritious snacks, using leftover bits of vegetables, nuts, fruits and seeds made up into robots, weirdos from the planet Boff!

Be careful not to overdo dried fruit – even the apparently safe ones can have an irritant effect on certain sensitive individuals. Hunza apricots are a particularly good buy.

Often you can persuade a reluctant vegetable eater by stir-frying chopped vegetables with chopped nuts, fruit and seeds. Select your cooking oil carefully and enhance the flavour of your cooking with herbs, fresh if possible.

When shopping don't be tempted into buying more than you really need; fresh items are best bought in smaller quantities to retain their quality. With fresh vegetables, if you buy a selection, seasonal ones are often cheaper; then keep as much as possible in the refrigerator, to retain maximum vitamin C levels. You will find costs will average themselves out, then when you've really got to grips with the budgetting a little treat of the more expensive varieties can be introduced to add a bit of style. The same ruling can be applied to fruit. In towns you might find that the major supermarkets have the pick of the quality; often disposing of produce classed as perishable at low prices. Take advantage of this and make sure that you are aware when their main turnover day is.

The various support groups do a grand job of keeping you up to date on new products on the market that are suitable; make sure that you take advantage of this and be prepared to send in any information you might come across, as every little bit can help.

Don't be downhearted by refusals to eat food, it might be a natural instinctive aversion. There are a number of different ways to cook foods, a variety of ways in which to dress them up and any number of combinations in which to mix and match. Even though it might seem a trifle unusual – try it; after all, think of some of the things pregnant women fancy or even expectant fathers!

Most people eat far more protein than they really need; if you reduce this and offset with an interesting and appetizing serving of vegetables you will find housekeeping bills levelling out without any serious detrimental effect to health.

The majority of people only have a few major restrictions on diet, but the things that are likely to give a substantial increase on your budgeting are the more unusual grains; this can be helped if you use a base of one of the cheaper flours that is low down on your allergy list. I have found that it is more likely the quantity of any given item that will increase the risk of allergy or intolerance rather than the frequency. Experience usually gives you an idea of how much you dare take at one go. If you have to buy organic produce, although it is unwise to assume that as you are allergic this could necessarily be beneficial (allergy can be set up to organic produce as well), then try and find someone who will deal with you direct. This might involve you in making up a little cooperative, as many organic growers are trying to make a profit and have to have a guaranteed viable outlet before putting your concerns before those of larger dealers. Bottled water is another major expense, and is becoming even more essential for many families, as normal water purity cannot be guaranteed. Some places are lucky enough to have it sold in fairly large quantities; most of us have to buy it in 2 Litre bottles. Try to select the water most suitable to your needs; some are more palatable than others, some have a predominance of minerals that perhaps are not particularly suitable to you and others do quite well – and if they are that bit cheaper they can be used for cookery purposes too.

Supplements might initially seem a major drain on resources, but if you average out the cost and think positive it doesn't seem nearly so bad. Perhaps you might be brave enough to try and seek the support of your local health authority on this!

Do find out from your local health shop exactly what is the extent of the range that they can supply; often they will try to stock other things if they know there is going to be a guaranteed sale – after all they are a business and the more they sell the more profit they make.

Find as many different wholesale lists as possible and peruse them at leisure, that way you find out exactly what is available. All too often we can be totally unfamiliar with what is currently available, simply because we didn't see it at the time that we were in the shop. Substitute sweetners are one of these kinds of items; a local supermarket could be selling one such at a competitive price. Maple syrup is an example that readily springs to mind, and if you didn't know of the existence of date syrup you wouldn't even ask for it.

All this could make a major difference as to whether you stick to the diet or not; in addition it will put you in with an even chance of winning the rest of the family over and there is nothing more complicated than having to provide several different meals, which places stress upon the cook and also creates a division within the family, which in turn can create a rift and make the patient more self conscious of his problems. Home should be a haven where you feel as much a harmonious part as possible. An illusion exists, that people with this kind of problem need sympathy because they cannot eat like everyone else; the truth of the matter is that they are very special, they get the best of everything, and so it really can't be that bad. What if they are not able to eat a bar of chocolate, are they really missing very much? After all, it is not essential to life and with the money saved a much more memorable treat can be had. Substitutes can always be found to counterbalance those times when the child feels the need to be like the others. If they are encouraged to share these things you regard as treats, they soon feel as much of the crowd as any other.

If the child or adult is going through a natural low period, (we can all become depressed no matter what our lifestyle is), this can be countered by emphasising the good points: 'Aren't you lucky, Tommy only gets beefburgers and chips, you get savoury nut burgers, Hawaiian salad and duchesse potatoes'. Invite people around to share an alternative meal (make sure it's one of your successes); it's surprising how persuasive a good meal can be.

Most people feel that they want to keep 'the problem' private because of the controversy and lack of general understanding on the subject. Do try to have the confidence to face up to this reticence; especially let anyone know who has major dealings with the sufferer. Provide a typewritten list of major problems that have to be faced up to, in a concise matter of fact way and make several copies, passing these on to the appropriate people, and keep one for yourself.

Persevere in getting your child's symptoms recognised by a reliable professional. I know of one particular incident where a mother was so distressed at the treatments her child had been forced to undergo, each person giving her a different opinion, that she sought private help and found out that the child had been suffering with milk allergy all the time, and just with a simple alteration in diet all the major symptoms disappeared.

If providing special food becomes a bone of contention, seek the help of your local community social worker or dietitian who will often help you find a way around this problem. Such people have good experience and knowledge about financial assistance available and how the different authorities work.

Eating out

Try to re-educate local groups dealing with children in your area to provide suitable alternative food and drink, as the numbers afflicted with this kind of problem are steadily growing. If not, arrange to bring a substitute; remember it's not your child's fault that he or she cannot eat certain foods, it's just something that confers special needs.

Arrange with the hostess prior to a party to have the things your child can eat on readily identifiable plates. Ask if the things that have been brought along can be put on their plates while everybody is tucking into their own. If people are busy feeding they rarely take much notice of what is going on around them. Find out what kind of foods are going to be on offer at the party; if jelly and ice cream, there are a variety of substitutes on the market that can be prepared beforehand: homemade jellies with carrageen or agar, and yoghourts can be made into a passable ice cream. There are a wide variety of alternative yoghourts now available – goats', ewes', soya – always check the ingredients. Always pack something that is enjoyed for eating out, then it can never be a disappointment. Often they come home having shared it with the others and feeling perfectly happy.

Teach children that being food sensitive is just something that you have to learn to live with like having bad eyesight or a larger than average nose!

Restaurants can seem to be a problem, but if you approach the family run type and explain the situation, they will often let you have unusual combinations not listed, or even let you add your own extras. I have no trouble getting an empty glass supplied to put spring water in, or getting a plate of vegetables only supplied. These occasional trips out boost morale even if you don't find it particularly exciting. I find the cost more limiting than the problem of the food.

Holidaying can seem a bit more daunting, but if you hunt around and are not afraid to ask, you find many people are sympathetic and usually an agreement can be worked out. I take a selection of suitable foods with me and have been known to join in on the cooking as I find people are very willing to find out how to prepare different foods, as they never know when it might be needed again. I assess beforehand, by letter, the scope in variety in the local shops, as the food shops are usually one of the first ports of call when arriving.

Tap-water can be a problem to some children. Apart from bottled spring water there are home filters which use granular activated charcoal to remove impurities. The initial cost of these is high but over 2 or 3 years it is much cheaper to buy a good filter than gallons of bottled water.

Bath-water can be treated with a small amount of bath salts, washing soda or a special kind of seasalt available at health stores. Time spent in the water should be limited. After swimming in a swimming bath shower well and rub a thin coating of unrefined cooking oil into the skin. Prior to swimming a course of homeopathic chlorum (6c) can be given as tablets and topped up each time beforehand. Some have found this helpful.

Finally

Don't expect miracles to happen overnight, a slow steady recovery is far more reliable. Flow with the tide as there are good times and bad times on the road to recovery.

Encourage a positive outlook. Don't dwell on the things that can't be done, concentrate energies into what can be. Develop hobbies and interests.

Try to interest others in your alternative eating habits as it can be fun for everyone.

Keep a record of positive improvements.

Don't attempt anything too complicated at first as far as diet goes; work out a base of safe, reliable recipes to work on.

Increase the positive odds in your favour i.e. could be moody because clothing is too tight or the fabric is irritating.

Look into the possible use of – Tissue Salts – Herbal remedies – to cope with minor problems; all too often with the allergic person it's the minor things that get out of hand.

Do not become obsessed with trying to do the right thing. What you are trying to do is encourage a gentle adaptation within your family lifestyle.

Seek out the appropriate support group that is suitable to your needs. These support groups are not government aided – everyone gives their time and effort voluntarily. Monies paid into such organisations give you much needed information and supports others who are trying to further the cause. The majority of people who write to these charities are part of the ever growing statistics that are never ever included on the government's official statistics. That does not mean that they don't exist and it certainly doesn't mean that their problems aren't as real as those that have been accounted for.

Think positively because that is the only way that this problem can be tackled and resolved.

Index